What is

sing?

nd Practice

Transforming Nursing Practice series

Transforming Nursing Practice is the first series of books designed to help students meet the requirements of the NMC Standards and Essential Skills Clusters for degree programmes. Each book addresses a core topic, and together they cover the generic knowledge required for all fields of practice. Accessible and challenging, *Transforming Nursing Practice* helps nursing students prepare for the demands of future healthcare delivery.

Core knowledge titles:

Series editor: Dr Shirley Bach, Head of the School of Nursing and Midwifery at the University of Brighton

Communication and Interpersonal Skills in Nursing (2nd edn)	ISBN 978 0 85725 449 8
Contexts of Contemporary Nursing (2nd edn)	ISBN 978 1 84445 374 0
Health Promotion and Public Health for Nursing Students	ISBN 978 0 85725 437 5
Introduction to Medicines Management in Nursing	ISBN 978 1 84445 845 5
Law and Professional Issues in Nursing (2nd edn)	ISBN 978 1 84445 372 6
Leadership, Management and Team Working in Nursing	ISBN 978 0 85725 453 5
Learning Skills for Nursing Students	ISBN 978 1 84445 376 4
Medicines Management in Adult Nursing	ISBN 978 1 84445 842 4
Medicines Management in Children's Nursing	ISBN 978 1 84445 470 9
Medicines Management in Mental Health Nursing	ISBN 978 0 85725 049 0
Nursing Adults with Long Term Conditions	ISBN 978 0 85725 441 2
Nursing and Collaborative Practice (2nd edn)	ISBN 978 1 84445 373 3
Nursing and Mental Health Care	ISBN 978 1 84445 467 9
Passing Calculations Tests for Nursing Students	ISBN 978 1 84445 471 6
Patient and Carer Participation in Nursing	ISBN 978 0 85725 307 1
Successful Practice Learning for Nursing Students (2nd edn)	ISBN 978 0 85725 315 6
What is Nursing? Exploring Theory and Practice (2nd edn)	ISBN 978 0 85725 445 0

Personal and professional learning skills titles:

Series editors: Dr Mooi Standing, Principal Lecturer/Enterprise Quality Manager in the Department of Nursing and Applied Clinical Studies, Canterbury Christ Church University and Dr Shirley Bach, Head of the School of Nursing and Midwifery at the University of Brighton

Clinical Judgement and Decision Making in Nursing	ISBN 978 1 84445 468 6
Critical Thinking and Writing for Nursing Students	ISBN 978 1 84445 366 5
Evidence-based Practice in Nursing	ISBN 978 1 84445 369 6
Information Skills for Nursing Students	ISBN 978 1 84445 381 8
Reflective Practice in Nursing	ISBN 978 1 84445 371 9
Succeeding in Research Project Plans and Literature Reviews for Nursing Students	ISBN 978 0 85725 264 7
Successful Professional Portfolios for Nursing Students	ISBN 978 0 85725 457 3
Understanding Research for Nursing Students	ISBN 978 1 84445 368 9

To order, contact our distributor: BEBC Distribution, Albion Close, Parkstone, Poole, BH12 3LL. Telephone: 0845 230 9000, email: learningmatters@bebc.co.uk. You can also find more information on each of these titles and our other learning resources at www.learningmatters. co.uk. Many of these titles are also available in various e-book formats, please visit our website for more information.

What is Nursing?

Exploring Theory and Practice

Second Edition

Carol Hall
Dawn Ritchie

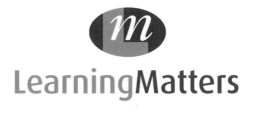

LearningMatters

First published in 2009 by Learning Matters Ltd

Second edition published 2011

British Library Cataloguing in Publication Data

A CIP record for this book is available from the British Library

ISBN: 978 0 85725 445 0

This book is also available in the following ebook formats:

Adobe ebook ISBN: 978 0 85725 447 4
ePUB ebook ISBN: 978 0 85725 446 7
Kindle ISBN: 978 0 85725 448 1

Cover and text design by Toucan Design
Project management by Diana Chambers
Typeset by Kelly Winter
Printed and bound in Great Britain by Short Run Press, Exeter, Devon

Learning Matters Ltd
20 Cathedral Yard
Exeter EX1 1HB
Tel: 01392 215560
E-mail: info@learningmatters.co.uk
www.learningmatters.co.uk

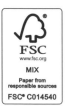

Contents

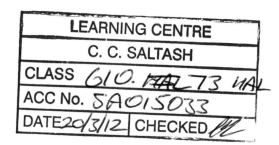
	Foreword	vi
	About the authors	vii
	Acknowledgements	viii
	Introduction	1
1	What is a nurse? The development of the nursing role	5
2	Being a professional nurse: image and values in nursing	26
3	Theories of nursing, and nursing as a caring activity	50
4	The nursing process	73
5	Nursing as a global health activity	98
6	Being qualified	119
7	Exploring the world of nursing by those working in it	143
	References	183
	Index	192

Foreword

This is a thoughtful and interesting, but most of all practical book, about what it really means to be a nurse. Beginning with a comparison of different definitions of nursing, the authors agree that nursing can be defined differently in diverse settings. They establish that all nursing is, however, influenced by the external effects of changes in society and social reform. They also explain the importance of funding, resources and changing healthcare policy.

The authors delve theoretically and philosophically into what we understand by the term 'being professional', such as the concepts of core values, and the scope and quality of being professional. This leads to a timely discussion on the contemporary images and stereotypes of nurses and nursing students.

One of the many useful facets of this book is the approach taken to applying and understanding nursing theory. Painting pen portraits of major theorists brings this into sharp relief. This emphasis continues by exploring the nurse's role in health promotion and nursing care through integrating what is being learned in the book into examples of what a nurse does. Practical frameworks are used to identify and manage nursing care problems in an accessible and supportive style.

In a creative departure from the usual nursing texts, the authors demonstrate how students can take the opportunity to learn about nursing in other cultures by widening horizons through electives and exchanges. If nursing and healthcare in the twenty-first century must embrace the global concept of health, and the effects of globalisation on worldwide health, what better way is there to understand this than through experiencing healthcare beyond the borders of the UK?

The final part of the book concentrates on life after being a student and the real world of working as a nurse. Again, this takes a refreshing departure from other nursing texts and provides excellent advice, tips and underpinning research on life as a newly qualified nurse. The value of pre-ceptorship and techniques for adapting to being qualified are covered here. The book provides advice on preparing for employment as a qualified nurse – for example, tips on interviewing and finding employment.

The authors explore the real world of working in nursing with detailed commentary from qualified nurses on what it is like to work in the four fields of nursing. This will provide invaluable help for students to plan for their future roles and career options. This book clearly demonstrates what nursing is, and can be, and that learning to be a nurse and qualifying is not the end of a process, but the beginning of a fulfilling and challenging, ever changing profession.

Shirley Bach
Series Editor

About the authors

Dr Carol Hall is an Associate Professor at the School of Nursing, University of Nottingham. She enjoys teaching practical elements of nursing within pre-registration nursing curricula, as well as supervising pre- and post-registration students in their dissertations and theses. She has a background in Children's Nursing and Nursing Education.

Dawn Ritchie is a Lecturer in Child Health Nursing at the University of Nottingham. She has been involved in nurse education for a number of years, including pre-registration and learning beyond registration programmes, and has developed a keen interest in the practical application of nursing. Dawn's clinical background is in critical and acute care in children's nursing.

Contributors

Valerie Gorton is Principal Lecturer and International Coordinator at the Institute of Health and Society, University of Worcester.

Gill Langmack is a Lecturer in Nursing at the University of Nottingham. Involved principally in pre-registration curricula, she enjoys developing practical ways of learning embracing new technologies to expand students' knowledge and skills. Her background is in critical care and acute children's nursing.

Acknowledgements

The authors and publisher are grateful to the following for their help in preparing this book:

- Dr Shirley Bach, series editor, for her advice for how best to update the first edition in the light of the most recent developments in nursing education;
- Liz Aston, Justine Barksby, Karen Billyeald, Louise Cook, Paula Dawson, Anne Felton, Bob Hallawell, Sheila Rose, Helen Saxelby, Gemma Stacey and Theo Stickley for their input into the final chapter.
- *The Nursing Standard*, for permission to reproduce the spider diagram 'The desired core values of nursing', as Figure 2.1 on page 31.

Introduction

Welcome to *What is Nursing?* This book aims to offer you a clear introduction to nursing from practical, professional and theoretical perspectives, as well as the reality of 'insider' understanding and experiences of what being a nurse means today. The chapters have been written by registered nurses working in nursing education with students, and in nursing practice caring for patients and clients. It has an approachable style, and aims to give you helpful information and learning opportunities as you move towards the profession of nursing, through the use of concept and research summaries, case studies and activities. Whether you are wondering what being a nurse is like and are thinking about applying to university, or are already on a nursing course, or even about to qualify, this book will have something for you.

The early chapters of the book focus on understanding what contemporary nursing is, and how it developed as a profession. They also explore ideas such as understanding your newly developing role and practice as a nurse with the patients and clients in your care.

The later chapters address topics such as globalisation and international working, becoming qualified and the practical roles of qualified nurses. Although these may seem to be mostly of interest to nurses who are nearing registration or who are undertaking work abroad, they also offer a clear illustration of what it is like to be a nurse in these situations. For those of you who are new nursing students, or planning to become a member of our profession, having such an opportunity for a sneak preview into the world of qualified practice may inspire. Certainly, such an opportunity allows considerations of some very real challenges and the chance to think about these comfortably and safely in your own time before arriving as a newly qualified practitioner.

Activities and other learning features

You can read this book from cover to cover if you wish. However, it is primarily a learning environment – with specific features to help you learn and think for yourself. At various stages within each chapter there are points at which you can break to undertake activities. Undertaking and understanding the activities is an important element of your understanding of the content of each chapter. You are encouraged, where appropriate, to reflect on your practice and consider how the things you have learned from working with patients might inform your understanding of clinical judgement and decision making. Other activities will require you to take time away from the book to find out new information that will add to your understanding of the topic under discussion. Some activities challenge you to apply your learning to a question or scenario to help you reflect on issues and practice in more depth. A few activities require you to make observations during your day-to-day life or in the clinical setting. All these activities are designed to increase your understanding of the topics under discussion and how they reflect on nursing practice.

Where appropriate, there are suggested or potential answers to activities at the end of the chapter. It is recommended that you try where possible to engage with the activities in order to increase your understanding of the realities of twenty-first century nursing.

There are also concept and research summaries, as well as other reminders of important ideas or definitions, which give you evidence and sometimes offer extra opportunities to further your knowledge and understanding with sources outside the book.

Overview of chapters

Chapter 1 aims to introduce you to nursing by helping you to develop your knowledge about how nursing has been defined and developed as a modern profession. You are challenged to think about how you perceive nursing today, and also to think about nursing in light of historical development. You will explore the way nursing has changed as the result of legal and professional regulation. You are encouraged to think about your own views and values in respect of nursing work, as you begin to engage with, and commit to, the principles of becoming a nurse.

The focus in Chapter 2 moves from the profession of nursing to exploring the image and role of the professional nurse. You are invited to explore key features of what makes a professional identity in nursing and consider the evolution of contemporary images and representations of nursing. You are challenged to think about your values concerning the nurse as a professional, and consider how professional values are set down within *The Code: Standards of Conduct, Performance and Ethics for Nurses and Midwives* (NMC, 2008a), and the *Guidance on Professional Conduct for Nursing and Midwifery Students* (NMC, 2009a). The professional role of the nurse will be discussed in respect of care for patients, clients and carers, and also other healthcare professionals across a breadth of settings where nursing care is delivered.

In Chapter 3 you will explore the nurse's caring and therapeutic relationships with patients and clients by examining a number of theoretical ideas about nursing. Nursing as an evidence-based participative activity is introduced and you will explore how nursing activity is constructed, the way that you understand nursing roles and the way in which roles of clients do impact on the way you will deliver care. This is illustrated for you as well as challenging you to think about developing your own examples. Thinking and doing is a core theme in this chapter.

Chapter 4 takes the thinking and doing theme much further. You will consider the 'tools of the trade' for nurses. In this chapter, systematic processes of nursing are identified and you are challenged to think about the way that you might assess client needs and plan, deliver and evaluate the care that you give and determine the effectiveness for recipients. It is essential in nursing to ensure that care given is recorded, so this chapter encourages you to develop your skills in writing and recording information effectively, and to determine measures by which outcomes can be established. The chapter develops your thinking much more about how your knowledge is needed in order to be able to nurse effectively and looks in more detail at the role of evidence in delivering best practice. Finally, to work effectively you must manage your care within a wider team and this can be arranged in many ways. You are encouraged to think about different approaches to care delivery taken across a variety of care settings.

Nursing and healthcare in the twenty-first century must embrace the global concept of health and the effects of globalisation on worldwide health and Chapter 5 encourages you to widen your knowledge of nursing from the UK to the wider world. You are able to explore opportunities available to develop and enhance your cultural knowledge and experiences, particularly in respect of nursing in other countries and with other cultures. You will be introduced to material that will assist you to explore your knowledge, values and beliefs in relation to global health issues.

Chapter 6 looks specifically at what it is like to qualify as a nurse at the end of a nurse education course within a higher education institution. What are the worries and concerns newly qualified nurses have, and how can the various initiatives available help make the transition to a qualified, skilled and practising nurse a smooth one? The chapter works with you to think about getting a job and what it is like to be a qualified nurse and how the role differs from being a student. You are also guided to think about mentoring students and what this is like.

In Chapter 7, the final and unique chapter of our book, excerpts from group interviews with nurses are used to offer you a real illustration of nursing work in all the main fields of practice in the UK – learning disability, children's, mental health and adult nursing. The nurses talking in the interviews currently work in a range of careers within these fields of practice and share their experiences with you, in order to enable you to understand their work and the benefits (and sometimes challenges) of being a nurse. The aim of the chapter is to help you understand the roles and practices of these nurses in their work and to explore, from their perspective, what it is like to be a qualified nurse today. It is not pretended that the sections will cover every element of nursing practice in each field of practice; indeed, that would be impossible to achieve. However, the aim is to address some key and representative elements of practice and give a flavour of the values and concerns of the profession.

NMC *Standards for Pre-registration Nursing Education* and Essential Skills Clusters

The Nursing and Midwifery Council (NMC) has standards of competence that have to be met by applicants to different parts of the nursing and midwifery register. These standards are what the NMC deems as necessary for the delivery of safe, effective nursing practice. As well as specific competencies, the NMC identifies specific skills that nursing students must have at various points of their training programme. These Essential Skills Clusters (ESCs) are essential abilities that students need to attain in order to practise to their full potential.

This book identifies some of the competencies and skills, within the realm of clinical judgement and decision making that student nurses need in order to be entered on to the NMC register. These competencies and ESCs are presented at the start of each chapter so that it is clear which of them the chapter addresses. All of the competencies and ESCs in this book relate to the *generic standards* that all nursing students must achieve. This book includes the latest taken from the *Standards for Pre-registration Nursing Education* (NMC, 2010).

Chapter 1
What is a nurse? The development of the nursing role

Carol Hall

NMC Standards for Pre-registration Nursing Education

As this chapter is concerned with defining contemporary nursing, it will use the generic standards for competence as a baseline.

Domain 1: Professional values

All nurses must act first and foremost to care for and safeguard the public. They must practise autonomously and be responsible and accountable for safe, compassionate, person-centred, evidence-based nursing that respects and maintains dignity and human rights. They must show professionalism and integrity and work within recognised professional, ethical and legal frameworks. They must work in partnership with other health and social care professionals and agencies, service users, their carers and families in all settings, including the community, ensuring that decisions about care are shared.

Domain 2: Communication and interpersonal skills

All nurses must use excellent communication and interpersonal skills. Their communications must always be safe, effective, compassionate and respectful. They must communicate effectively using a wide range of strategies and interventions including the effective use of communication technologies. Where people have a disability, nurses must be able to work with service users and others to obtain the information needed to make reasonable adjustments that promote optimum health and enable equal access to services.

Domain 3: Nursing practice and decision making

All nurses must practise autonomously, compassionately, skilfully and safely, and must maintain dignity and promote health and wellbeing. They must assess and meet the full range of essential physical and mental health needs of people of all ages who come into their care. Where necessary they must be able to provide safe and effective immediate care to all people prior to accessing or referring to specialist services irrespective of their field of practice. All nurses must also meet more complex and coexisting needs for people in their own nursing field of practice, in any setting including hospital, community and at home. All practice should be informed by the best available evidence and comply with local and national guidelines. Decision making must be shared with service users, carers and families

continued overleaf . . .

continued . . .

and informed by critical analysis of a full range of possible interventions, including the use of up-to-date technology. All nurses must also understand how behaviour, culture, socio-economic and other factors, in the care environment and its location, can affect health, illness, health outcomes and public health priorities and take this into account in planning and delivering care.

Domain 4: Leadership, management and team working

All nurses must be professionally accountable and use clinical governance processes to maintain and improve nursing practice and standards of healthcare. They must be able to respond autonomously and confidently to planned and uncertain situations, managing themselves and others effectively. They must create and maximise opportunities to improve services. They must also demonstrate the potential to develop further management and leadership skills during their period of preceptorship and beyond.

Chapter aims

After reading this chapter, you will be able to:

- define nursing from your own understanding and from existing theoretical perspectives;
- understand how nursing has developed as a modern profession and how it is changing today;
- outline some key historical and legislative guidance, and show how it has impacted on the contemporary definition of nursing;
- provide a professional definition of nursing.

Introduction

This chapter will help you to develop your knowledge about how nursing has been defined and developed as a modern profession. It will challenge you to think of how nursing is perceived by you and by others in light of history and how nursing has emerged in relation to the way it is defined today. You will also be able to explore examples of the way nursing has developed as the result of legal and professional regulation. This will help you to be aware of the implications of regulation in nursing, as well as reflect on your own views and values, as you begin to engage with, and commit to, the principles of becoming a nurse. Finally, you will be introduced to material that will consider your role as a nurse in promoting health and in nursing the sick person. There will be an opportunity to explore nursing across a range of patients, including adults, children, those with mental health concerns and individuals who have special learning needs, which may result in a requirement for nursing and social care.

This chapter is intended to underpin and provide context for the remaining chapters of the book, so it is important to expect to see reference made to elements to be found in later chapters. You can follow these references immediately if you wish, in order to develop a specific area of learning, or view them as indicators and return to them later.

Defining nursing: what do you think?

Nursing may not be easy to describe, but patients know when they get good nursing and when they do not. Nursing requires a high level set of skills and understanding which taken separately may seem commonplace and undemanding but combined as a whole is far more complex and powerful.
(Christine Beasley, Chief Nursing Officer for England (DH, 2006, p4))

In exploring definitions of nursing it is essential to consider your own perspectives and allow these to form part of the context of your thinking. Like the patients described by Beasley (2006) above, it is reasonable to assume that you already have some views from your life experience of what may define a nurse. This chapter will, therefore, begin with your own ideas and then use this backdrop to start comparing the thinking of others.

Activity 1.1   *Research and evidence-based practice*

The Department of Health for the UK employs a team of advisers who consider all areas of nursing and healthcare. The Chief Nursing Officer (CNO) is the Government's most senior nursing adviser. In England, the CNO has responsibility for delivering the Government's strategy for nursing and leads nearly 600,000 nurses, midwives and health visitors and allied health professionals (DH, 2007a). There are also CNOs for Scotland, Wales and Northern Ireland.

Look up the CNO's page on the Department of Health Website: **www.dh.gov.uk/en/ Aboutus/Chiefprofessionalofficers/Chiefnursingofficer/index.htm**

Make a note of any recent topics or correspondence accessible from this page. What appear to you to be the most pressing issues for nurses today?

As what you find will depend on topical developments, there is no outline answer at the end of the chapter.

Activity 1.2 will enable you to start exploring nursing definitions from your own perceptions. The definition that you create will be referred to as you progress through the chapter and you will be able to develop your own ideas. It may be useful to consider this work for inclusion in your professional portfolio.

Activity 1.2   *Reflection*

From what you already know, think about how you might define a nurse and jot down your own ideas.

Now look at your notes – reflect over the following.

- How did you try to define nursing?
- What do you already know and how has this influenced you?
- Did you try to identify what nurses do, for example 'they care for people'?
- Did you try to identify nurses by what they know, for example 'they know about medications' or by their image or attitude or behaviour, for example 'they wear a uniform', 'they are professional'?

As this activity is based on your own reflection, there is no outline answer at the end of the chapter.

You are now beginning to consider the same issues as have been preoccupying some very eminent nurses for many years, and the above exercises may have shown you that nursing is complex and difficult to define. In respect of having a unique body of knowledge usually associated with a profession, this is even more difficult.

Nursing is influenced by where it happens, who is being nursed and by the resources that might be needed and the availability of these. In this chapter, we will explore how nursing is portrayed and defined as the result of existing knowledge around nursing. How nursing as a profession is perceived is also influenced by image and by experience, and these elements will be addressed in more detail in the next chapter. The concept of nursing as a profession will be addressed too. Nursing is finally defined by beliefs and this will be addressed in more detail in Chapter 3, where values, philosophies and models around delivering nursing are considered in more depth.

Why is having a clear definition of nursing important?

Defining nursing is essential for a number of reasons, and these are succinctly summarised in the Royal College of Nursing (RCN, 2003) document *Defining Nursing*, where the following reasons for a definition of nursing are identified. A definition of nursing enables nurses to:

- describe nursing to people who do not understand it;
- clarify their role in the multidisciplinary healthcare team;
- influence the policy agenda at local and national level;
- develop educational curricula;
- identify areas where research is needed to strengthen the knowledge base of nursing;
- inform decisions about whether and how nursing work should be delegated to other personnel;

- support negotiations at local and national level on issues such as nurse staffing, skill mix and nurses' pay.
  (Adapted from RCN, 2003, p4)

Activity 1.3   *Critical thinking*

Take a critical look at the RCN summary document *Defining Nursing*, which can be found at **www.rcn.org.uk.**

Examine the different definitions that are outlined within it and consider the following questions.

- Do you agree with the final statement that is drawn?
- Does the paper describe nursing for everyone?
- Are there any limitations of this definition?

After reading this paper, try to think of how you would now describe nursing to a friend who does not know what it is. Jot down your ideas in about 5–6 key words. Have your original ideas changed?

As this activity is based on your own reflection, there is no outline answer at the end of the chapter.

Concept summary: What is the Royal College of Nursing?

The Royal College of Nursing (RCN) is a UK-wide 'professional organisation' for nursing. This means it is a non-profit-making membership organisation that seeks to further the profession of nursing and act in supporting its members in their relationships with employers. The RCN develops professional documents and journals for nursing, arranges conferences to share nursing knowledge, and consults members to lobby the Government, and other organisations, to improve nursing. It also works with the International Council of Nurses (ICN) and the World Health Organization (WHO) to represent UK interests in the global nursing arena. The RCN also acts as a union for its members. Unite/Amicus and UNISON are also trade unions that represent nurses. For more information on all these organisations, visit **www.rcn.org.uk**, **www.icn.ch**, **www.who.int**, **www.unison.org** and **www.amicustheunion.org**.

It is important to recognise that the RCN is not the only group that has tried to define nursing, and while *Defining Nursing* makes a useful contribution to British thinking, nursing is carried out globally and it is important to think of nursing across countries as well as within them. The RCN's ideals are identified as being commensurate with a wider definition of nursing globally, which is addressed by the International Council of Nurses (ICN):

Nursing encompasses autonomous and collaborative care of individuals of all ages, families, groups and communities, sick or well and in all settings. Nursing includes the promotion of health, prevention of illness and the care of ill, disabled and dying people. Advocacy, promotion of a safe environment, research, participation in shaping health policy, and in patient and health systems management, and education are also key nursing roles. (ICN, 2010)

For the purposes of this book, the above definition will be used, because it clearly includes some of the elements of nursing that the NMC wants to ensure you develop and these are addressed more explicitly than in the RCN definition. It is also a useful tool when considering European and international nursing in Chapter 6 of this book. However, the RCN definition and those of others in the UK are commensurate and compatible with the ICN definition.

The role of regulators in defining nursing

The Nursing and Midwifery Council (NMC) was established in accordance with UK law under The Nursing and Midwifery Order 2001(SI 2002/253) (HM Government, 2002) and came into existence on 1 April 2002, taking over from a previous regulatory body known as the United Kingdom Central Council for Nursing and Midwifery (UKCC).

The NMC is a 'professional regulator' for nursing. This means that it acts to safeguard the health and well-being of the public by regulating, reviewing and promoting nursing and midwifery standards. The NMC is monitored by the Charity Commission and by the Council for Healthcare Regulatory Excellence (CHRE).

To achieve its aims, the NMC (2010b):

- maintains a register of all nurses and midwives and ensure that they are properly qualified and competent to work in the UK;
- sets the standards of education, training and conduct that nurses and midwives need to deliver high quality healthcare consistently throughout their careers;
- ensures that nurses and midwives keep their skills and knowledge up to date and uphold the standards of their professional code;
- ensures that midwives are safe to practise by setting rules for their practice and supervision;
- has fair processes to investigate allegations made against nurses and midwives who may not have followed the code.

You should note that, in addition to formal definitions of nursing, as the regulator of nurses in the UK, the NMC also has positions on the way that nurses are prepared for practice and on the roles that nurses play. This will be addressed much more thoroughly in relation to the concept of a professional included in Chapter 2. However, it should be recognised that the regulators have a defining concern with what nurses do, in ensuring safe, high-quality and ethically sound care for the public once registered, rather than being concerned with a definition of nursing in its broader sense.

The NMC translates the broader definitions of nursing into the practicalities of what nurses must do through identified standards for professional practice. These include the NMC *Standards for*

Pre-registration Nursing Education (NMC, 2010) which outline proficiencies for achievement in order to register. The NMC has also identified Essential Skills Clusters (ESCs) for nursing (NMC, 2010) which address very particularly what nursing students completing pre-registration programmes within the UK must be assessed as doing safely in order to register.

Activity 1.4   *Research and reflection*

Put yourself in the NMC's position for a moment – what do you think would be 'essential' skills for all nurses to learn?

Now use the NMC website (**www.nmc.org.uk**) to identify the skills you will need to learn in order to achieve the ESCs as prescribed by the NMC.

*   Do these match what you thought about?
*   Are there any more essential skills you think should be included as well as these?
*   Do they help to define what nurses should do?

As this activity is based on your own reflection, there is no outline answer at the end of the chapter.

How the law defines nursing

Nursing also has to meet some defining criteria established by law. This includes both national and international statute, and there may be variance in definitions across and between countries in order to accommodate national law.

National law has three major purposes: that of professional regulation as defined above in relation to the NMC; that of civil or common law (tort) related to ensuring a duty to care; and finally that of criminal law in enforcing legally acceptable behaviour by nurses.

Concept summary: Criminal law and civil law – what is the difference?

Civil law

This is legislation that is used to settle disputes; i.e., it is used to claim for damages. The claimant is the person or body who has been 'harmed' and the defendant is the person or body who has to prove that they were not liable for the harm caused. The outcome of a successful civil case may be payment of damages by the defendant or an injunction against them. Civil law is applicable to all instances that involve patient care. If you are an employer you may also be liable for any harm that may come to your staff while they are in your employment.

Criminal law

This is legislation that is used by the state to enforce behaviour; i.e., it is legislation that, if contravened, generally results in the state becoming the prosecutor and a defendant, if found guilty, receiving either imprisonment, a community penalty or a fine.

(Adapted from McHale and Tingle, 2007, pp2–3)

All nurses (and indeed all health carers) have a duty of care to their patients that upholds the rights of patients to receive care from nurses that is carried out appropriately by personnel who have the skills to perform care safely and effectively.

But what is meant by 'safely' and 'effectively'? It is often hard when you go into practice to work out what you can do and what you cannot. This is especially so when you are new to nursing as a student. While many other influences might dictate whether or not you can or cannot do different aspects of practice (local policies, your mentor's guidance, your university's rules), in law, the consideration of this definition of nursing is much wider. Specific tasks (such as whether you can collect a patient from the operating theatre) are not included, but they are addressed broadly in identifying that, if you carry out an activity, then you must be competent to do so. The main points of civil law relate mostly to what might be considered as negligence.

Cox (2006) identifies that if, as you perform your work as a nurse, things go wrong, in a court of law you would be judged against the standard reasonably expected from any other ordinarily competent nurse carrying out that particular task. No excuse can be made for inexperience, because if you cannot carry out the task, you should not take it on and, further, your mentor or employer should not let you. This does not suggest, however, that your mentor or employer is entirely accountable for your actions. While they do make decisions about delegating nursing tasks and hold some accountability for this, you have an accountability too in taking the task on in the first place under the duty of care for your patient. Further, you must carry out any care you give to a reasonable standard, and there is no excuse for poor basic standards that compromise the quality or safety of care given.

In respect of criminal law, nurses have a duty to be law-abiding and this means being aware of the legal requirements of being a British citizen generally. When you qualify as a nurse, the NMC requires your university to declare your honesty and integrity, thus identifying that, in their opinion, you are a suitable person to enter the profession. During your time on a nursing course, you must also develop your own understanding of a wide range of legislation as it applies to nursing. You will be introduced to the law and the many ways it defines your roles as a nurse as you go through your programme of study, but here is a short case study to get you started in your thinking.

Scenario

You go to a practice learning experience in an acute mental health setting. Here you observe nurses working with a client who is assessed as requiring admission for treatment, but who wants to go home. He is becoming increasingly agitated and upset, and is threatening to walk out. He begins to abuse the nurses verbally, shouting loudly and shaking his fists at them. The nurses work to help the client through effective communication and through facilitating the patient's self-administration of prescribed medication.

The laws that define nursing in the situation shown in this scenario are many, and are both criminal and civil. Here are some – and you may think of more. The client may need to be admitted under the requirements of the Mental Health Act and must therefore stay in the care setting. The nurse has a duty of care to the client to ensure that the care given is safe and of a quality deemed to be of a standard expected of a competent practitioner, and this will include ensuring the client's safety. The client's aggression towards the nurses is unacceptable and may breach criminal law if it is deemed to be assault. The nurses must assess the situation in relation to the Health and Safety Executive (HSE), which places a duty to report any incident that results in a dangerous occurrence under the Reporting of Injuries, Diseases and Dangerous Occurrences Regulations (1995) (RIDDOR). This would apply if the patient injured himself through trying to escape the situation or if the violence escalated and resulted in the nurses becoming severely injured, or injured to the extent that they were unfit to work for longer than three days. In order to give the medicinal treatment required, the nurses would need to work within the legal requirements of the Medicines Act (HM Government, 1968), Misuse of Drugs Act (HM Government, 1971) and the Misuse of Drugs Regulations (HM Government, 1985). They would be following professional guidance from the NMC and also their local medicines policy. If the nurses did not follow local policy, their employers would not be expected to take any liability for their actions if anything went wrong.

Activity 1.5 — Research and evidence-based practice

Go to the HSE website – **www.hse.gov.uk** – and look for the page on RIDDOR.

Then answer the following questions.

* Who should report an incident at work?
* What sort of incidents should be reported?
* What is the ICC, and how would you contact it?
* What records of an incident and its reporting do you need to keep?

There is an outline answer to this activity at the end of the chapter.

The role of European legislation in defining a nurse

Finally for this section, the definition of a registered nurse across Europe is governed by European Union (EU) law through directives. These laws are agreed by the EU countries, including the UK. As an example in nursing, currently the UK agree governance in respect of European law under the EU Directive on Mutual Recognition of Professional Qualification (DIR 2005/36/EC) (EU, 2005). (This came into force in October 2007 and supersedes two previous EU directives in identifying the required time for nurse training and the broad areas of education and practice required.)

While the content in this directive currently applies only to those nurses undertaking the adult nursing field of practice in the UK, the NMC interprets the guidance in relation to the required number of hours that nurses need to work in order to register as being relevant for all nurses. According to the NMC (2010), to qualify for registration a period of study, including 2,300 hours of theory and 2,300 hours of practice, and not less than three years of education, must be undertaken to qualify to enter the register. This is important for universities who are designing programmes for nursing, but also identifies for you why your university may sometimes seem very strict about monitoring your attendance both in the university and in your practice placements. Because of the need to comply with the law and professional regulation relating to practice, nursing cannot allow students to miss practical or taught time from the course and learn in other ways, as perhaps may be acceptable in other university courses.

Understanding regulations is also particularly important in order for you to gain an appreciation of your future professional role and be able to discuss it in an informed way, as required by the NMC to achieve competencies by the second progression point (NMC, 2010). This is therefore going to be revisited and addressed further in relation to the concept of professionalism and the relationship between image and nursing.

How has history determined a contemporary consideration of nursing?

In order to unpack the definitions explored thus far, it is useful to consider a little about the way in which nursing has emerged historically, within the context of professional practice. British nursing has been shaped by factors both inside and outside the profession itself, and continues to be transformed by these influences. It is vital for you to understand and be able to discuss the impact and potential advantages and disadvantages of change resulting from these forces. Also, understanding the wider relationship between nursing and other care contexts, and how collaboration and close working interprofessionally can enhance nursing is equally important. The nature of these relationships is addressed in two other books in this series in detail, should you wish to consider these aspects more thoroughly (Goodman and Clemow, 2010; Williamson et al., 2010). This section merely serves as an introduction to this context.

Nursing is influenced by the external impact of societal need and social reform, by the availability of available funding and resources, and by changing healthcare policy, such as the development of the National Health Service (NHS). Political perceptions of nursing as both a profession and a workforce, indicated by NHS career structure reforms and by decisions over pay and the extension of roles in practice, are also influential as are changes in legal requirements, such as the European Working Time Directive (2003/88/EC), which has influenced the duration of time that nurses and their medical colleagues can be expected to work, thus leading to changes in working practice in order to maintain effective services for patients. Finally, changes in available workforce and workforce mobility are also influential. For example, changes in the EU and the increased mobility of new accession countries have led to contemporary workforce change in the UK nursing system. Between the years 2007 and 2008, the number of Romanian nurses in the UK increased significantly, while the number of overseas registrants fell due to changes in admission criteria (NMC 2007–2008).

Examples of internal forces include the identification of a need for regulation and qualification, changes in the work undertaken by nurses through innovation projects (such as clinical specialist roles and nurse-led clinics) and inter- and intra-hospital changes to improve or change patient service. This may include the transfer of service from acute to community, or from medical to nurse-led settings.

It is important to recognise, of course, that none of these considerations in principle is actually new, although the examples emerging may have changed. Forms of nursing activity alongside medicine have been identified in historical writing in the time of the Ancient Greeks and regularly in writings from this period onwards, according to classic work by Baly (1995).

It is, therefore, useful to consider the emergence of modern nursing through the contextual lens of earlier historical description. Looking at nursing this way enables some differentiation between activities that relate to nursing and the concept of the nurse as the professional we identify today.

This section of the chapter will explore the following key themes taken from the ICN definition of nursing presented earlier in the chapter. You will be able to consider how these have come to define nursing today using examples from an historical perspective.

- Nursing as autonomous and collaborative.
- Advocacy and the promotion of a safe environment as functions of nursing.
- Nursing and the development, transmission and application of evidence through research, policy management and education.

Nursing as autonomous and collaborative

Autonomy

Autonomy in nursing is defined as *the exercise of considered independent judgement to effect a desired outcome* (Keenan, 1999, p10).

<table>
<tr><td>

Activity 1.6   *Research and evidence-based practice*

</td></tr>
</table>

Activity 1.6 — Research and evidence-based practice

Ask yourself if you think nursing is an 'autonomous' activity today. Or is it dependent upon others for the care given to all individuals, sick or well, in all settings? Also, what might be the consequence of autonomy for the nurses, for patients and for other professionals?

Look up the article by Keenan (1999), A concept analysis of autonomy (*Journal of Advanced Nursing*, 29(3): 556–62), to help you to develop your thinking about autonomy in nursing.

Now read the next section and see whether your ideas are supported.

As this activity is based on your own reflection, and the answers to this are discussed in the text, there is no outline answer at the end of the chapter.

Historically, nursing dependence upon related professions is well documented, particularly in relation to nursing's relationship with medicine. However, it is nursing's interdependence with society and independence in professional terms that are equally relevant for exploration. It is clear from historical texts that the tending of the sick and the poor has developed in accordance with the needs of individual societies and continues to do so. While defining nursing at the level of the ICN is possible, the interpretation of such a definition varies from country to country, and is dependent upon the requirements and cultures of those societies at different times in history. An example of this can be seen in early nursing history in the UK. Consider the social change occurring in the late nineteenth century. At this time, there was a movement from a rural economy towards an increasingly industrialised society. This led to increasing urbanisation and healthcare changed to meet needs. Larger institutions for hospital treatment and care became more prevalent, with a corresponding move away from care offered by charitable or religious groups within local communities.

The impact of such change resulted in a provision of high-volume, poor-quality nursing activities with poor outcomes within workhouses. Eventually, this led to recognition of a need for professional development and ultimately regulation to ensure the quality of care delivery defined by 'qualified' nurses.

It is important, therefore, to identify that nursing does not operate within a vacuum, and the social and political context prevailing during the development and definition of nursing is also critical in determining an outcome. If you consider the wider context in the above historical situation, it is clear that nursing was not defined only by its own concerns. Towards the end of the nineteenth century, there was also ongoing sociopolitical change for women in the UK, related to the suffragette movement's demands for the right to vote and the need for recognition of greater rights generally for women. Women were looking for respectable career opportunities and a greater recognition, something offered by Florence Nightingale and others in the development of new nurse training schools. Later, during the First World War, as women took over roles in the absence of men at war, such opportunities became more visible. In 1919, after the end of the First World War, nursing was granted registration and with this the development of the foundation of modern nursing as an accountable and autonomous profession was cemented.

Throughout the time of history to the present day, it is possible to find examples of the influence of social policy on the development of the role of the nurse across all of the fields of practice.

Activity 1.7   *Critical thinking*

Identify a time period since the development of modern UK nursing following the requirement for registration in 1919 (you can choose any year). Try to find out what was happening in nursing and healthcare, and then look at the wider context of what was happening in the UK, and even around the world, at that time . . . what are the relationships? Did the definition of nursing change because of the situations and, if so, how?

Now think about nursing practice – did the patient experience change?

If you are from another country, you can use your own examples too.

If nursing did change, are those changes still visible in today's profession?

As this activity is based on your own reflections, there is no outline answer at the end of the chapter.

Collaboration in nursing

Collaboration in nursing can be defined as the way in which nurses work together and in partnership with others. This may be proactive, from a nurse's perspective, where a nurse sees a benefit to collaborate with others in order to achieve best practice, or it may be responsive to a wider position. In either of these, the number of potential collaborators in nursing is very large and will depend upon the care setting. Think about the examples in the case study below.

Case study: A distressed patient

Jane is an 89-year-old woman who has a fractured femur after being run over by a car near her home. She is going to have an operation tomorrow to secure the fracture. After her operation, Jane will be able to return home, but will need physiotherapy support and pain management care. Jane lives with her daughter in a small flat on the third floor of an apartment block. The nurse will need to collaborate with a range of other professionals in order to enable Jane to return home soon after her operation. This might include the occupational therapist and the physiotherapist, and also the main carer at home, who will be Jane's daughter.

Without proactive collaboration and discharge planning, Jane's needs for adequate pain relief, mobility and activity would not be met.

A further modern example regarding the nurse's responsive collaborative role relates to the costs of funding healthcare in the UK. The Skills for Health and Agenda for Change in this country have aims geared towards the breakdown of professional boundaries in healthcare and a drive towards greater flexibility in practices across roles. In practice, nurse leaders and workforce consultants use National Occupational Standards (NOS) to define a range of tasks. Collectively, these activities aim to define nursing roles in given situations. The tasks and outcomes can also be shared in part with other professions, and nursing can adopt new practices more usually associated with other professions. There has been a rise in non-medical prescribing, where nurses and other non-medical staff, including pharmacists, ophthalmologists and paramedics, can study to qualify to participate in prescribing – a role more conventionally undertaken by doctors.

For patients, this may offer better care more promptly and when it is needed. For example, the administration of statins by paramedics has meant much more rapid treatment for patients with myocardial infarction. This leads to a situation where greater collaboration is needed between professions to define who might carry out what activity and when. This type of responsive collaboration is critical in modern nursing and healthcare as roles change.

Concept summary: What are 'Skills for Health' and 'Agenda for Change'?

Skills for Health

Skills for Health was established to consider the roles and competences of all workers within the healthcare sector. The main strategic focus of Skills for Health is to develop a high quality, skilled, flexible and more productive workforce – for the whole sector in all UK nations – to raise the quality of health and healthcare for the public, patients and service users' (Skills for Health, Strategic Plan 2010–2015; 2009).

This has implications for all healthcare because Skills for Health does not focus on individual roles, but on the tasks that must be undertaken. Nursing cannot easily identify a unique body of skills, because nurses may not be the only people delivering these. It is the unique combination of skills and knowledge at a particularly defined level that may create the job description of a nurse. This system also enables services to move quickly in defining new roles and nurses may have to decide what they are prepared to undertake on an individual basis. It is conceivable that health carers of the future may include different professionals undertaking new roles.

For more information on Skills for Health, visit **www.skillsforhealth.org.uk/~/ media/Resource-Library/PDF/Strategic%20Plan%202010-15%20Mar%20 2010.ashx**

Agenda for Change

Agenda for Change is the NHS pay structure that is related closely to the Skills for Health arrangement. Established in 2004, Agenda for Change enables Trusts to decide the level of staff to be employed, and at what grade, in a nationally uniform manner across all nursing and allied healthcare workers' jobs. Agenda for Change uses a tool called the Knowledge and Skills Framework (KSF), which is closely linked to the professional development of nurses. These concepts are explored in relation to professionalism in Chapter 2.

For more information on Agenda for Change, visit **www.dh.gov.uk**.

The need to reduce the spiralling cost burden of the NHS is also paramount, and nurses' roles are likely to change in this climate. A modern example relates to the supportive health and social care provision made for elderly people in the UK. The issues around this population again are deeply contextualised in our social values and our politics.

In light of the National Health Service Act (HM Government, 1946), healthcare for all, free at point of delivery, was a promise made to citizens of the UK. This value of healthcare, free at point of delivery, has been sustained in principle since that time, but successes in the development of healthcare mean that a higher proportion of the population is living longer and requiring more treatment. Ultimately, this has forced some redefinition of what nursing care may be in modern times, because social care may require payment, while nursing care is provided within the NHS. Nursing has to collaborate with many others in the delivery of care and may share some skills with professionals whose prime role is social care, as well as those whose prime role is medicine, to give just two examples. However, nursing also must maintain clarity over the essence of practice that defines it uniquely in this shifting world.

Activity 1.8   *Decision making*

To explore this a little further you can review the parliamentary debates highlighted in the links below.

*   **www.publications.parliament.uk/pa/cm199900/cmselect/cmhealth/ 957/0110806.htm**
*   **www.publications.parliament.uk/pa/ld200001/ldhansrd/vo010322/ text/10322-29.htm**
*   **www.publications.parliament.uk/pa/ld200001/ldhansrd/vo010426/ text/10426-10.htm**

These relate to consideration of payment of elderly care in the community and in nursing homes in light of the Royal Commission on Long Term Care (DH, 1999) and the NHS Plan (DH, 2000), and have underpinned debate around the long-term funding of care that continues today (Glendinning, 2007). Look at where politicians have argued over the definition of nursing care in relation to the provision of care for the elderly. Follow this up by reading Ford et al.'s (2000) review of the importance of nursing definitions in this respect.

continued overleaf ...

continued . . . .

Ask yourself who stands to gain or lose in these discussions? How could clarity of definition help?

As this activity is based on your own observations and reflection, there is no outline answer at the end of the chapter.

In conclusion, contemporary nurses in the UK need to be clear in identifying distinct and clear boundaries in terms of a definition of the nursing profession, but at the same time must be confident in enabling an interpretation that allows the sharing of practical roles across professions in practice to offer the flexibility that service and patients require. In each setting where nursing occurs this may be interpreted differently, and this is especially the case for specialist nurses in particular areas of care. This concept establishes the ICN definition of the need for autonomous and collaborative practice.

Advocacy and the promotion of a safe environment as functions of nursing – historical considerations and contemporary comparison

The second feature of the ICN definition of nursing includes the role of the nurse as an advocate and as the promoter of a safe environment for patients. Although, on first review, these may seem to be strange companions in one statement, there are good reasons to explore them together. If you look at the work of Florence Nightingale, her consideration of nursing is a classical one, but it holds many lessons for today. Nightingale's model for nursing was one of both advocacy and of environmental manipulation. When you think about the historical and sociopolitical context, this view of nursing is not surprising and it makes sense.

Nightingale writes in *Notes on Hospitals* (1859) about the need for nurses to ensure that their patients have a clean, well-lit and well-ventilated environment, with separation to prevent the spread of infections. She identified the need to consider the patient's environment in promoting optimum return to health. The stringency of this approach, with consideration for the nurse's role in providing all aspects of basic care for the patient, amounted to a role for the nurse of advocating strongly for the achievement of better standards for all. Nursing was, however, emerging from a wider context of poor health standards in the population and there was a need for nurses to set an example in relation to health promotion. Further, there was limited opportunity for intervening to manage infection once it became established, as antibiotic treatment was not available. The requirement to manage and promote a healthy environment to enable a patient to return to full health was paramount. As an advocate for the patient, the nurse was expected to champion their patients' needs and educate them about their health.

In contemporary society this model of care still holds credence. Think about the incidences of infection in hospital today. *Clostridium difficile* (*C. diff.*), methicillin-resistant *Staphylococcus aureus* (*MRSA*) and *E. coli* are once again managed primarily through prevention. The use of care infection control and handwashing are major campaigns within the NHS (see **www.nhs.uk** and

www.rcn.org.uk). There is the recognition that prevention is better than cure, and the impact of resistance to antibiotic treatment has meant that widespread treatment is no longer considered beneficial. It is again recognised that prevention can be attained through the manipulation of the environment to create a safer place for patient care. This was also seen in community initiatives to prevent the spread of swine flu, which focused mainly on reducing the spread of infection. Patients and their families are also being educated to ensure that they question the care given and ask health carers whether they have washed their hands. This new (and yet old) approach to caring for patients once again recognises that the adaptation of nurses to the roles of health educator and advocate is a critical factor in keeping patients safe.

Activity 1.9   *Critical thinking*

Jason is three years old and cannot fight infection well by himself. He has just been diagnosed with a primary immune deficiency disorder.

- If you were Jason's nurse, what could you do to adapt the care environment to reduce his risk of getting an infection when he comes into hospital?
- How could you act as an advocate for Jason?
- In what ways could you offer health promotion to help Jason's family and his contacts?

Outline answers to this activity are given at the end of the chapter.

Nursing and the development, transmission and application of evidence through research, policy management and education

In operating in the best interests of the patient, nursing has a remit of providing the best care given existing knowledge and parameters. Nursing must also continually evaluate and appraise existing knowledge critically and develop new knowledge in order to look for new and better ways to care. In this definition of nursing, this means that nurses must be confident to question, critically and constructively, the existing knowledge they have and appraise their own work and that of others. Nurses should know how to use evidence effectively, and how to generate and develop evidence. To do this you will have to develop your skills of debate and discussion, and also begin to think critically when you are reading, watching, listening and thinking about your work.

Concept summary: But . . . what is critical appraisal?

A classic definition of critical thinking is by William Graham Sumner who described it as:

the examination and test of propositions of any kind which are offered for acceptance, in order to find out whether they correspond to reality or not. The critical faculty is a product of education and

> *training. It is a mental habit and power. It is a prime condition of human welfare that men and women should be trained in it. It is our only guarantee against delusion, deception, superstition, and misapprehension of ourselves and our earthly circumstances.*
> (Sumner, 1906, cited at **www.criticalthinking.org**)

Using Sumner's definition, it is important to realise that the habit of critical thinking is all around us. It is important to begin to get into the habit of questioning and then trying to answer those questions that you ask, if you can. A good place to start is by looking at the advertisements on television. Do you believe them? Do they define the product accurately? What may be the difficulty with the way the product is portrayed? The Advertising Standards Authority (ASA) is now responsible for ensuring the quality of advertisements, but in fact there are still many questions you may wish to ask.

Activity 1.10   *Critical thinking*

A good way for beginners to practise critical thinking is to turn to the daily newspapers. Try to read one or two very different ones that are relating the same story (for example, *The Guardian* and *Daily Mail* or *The Independent* and *The Sun*).

Compare the presentations of each. Are they saying the same or do they put a different presentation forward? If so, who do you believe and why? Try to think about your own perspectives as you begin to appraise the writing of others critically. What is your political perspective and what are your values?

When you feel confident with newspapers, try professional journals.

As this activity is based on your own observations and reflection, there is no outline answer at the end of the chapter.

Brookfield (1987) suggests that the components of critical thinking are:

- identifying and challenging assumptions;
- becoming aware of the importance of context in creating meaning;
- imagining and exploring alternatives;
- cultivating reflective scepticism.

In exploring nursing as a critically able professional, it is therefore important that you are able to raise questions and reflect on those questions. If you are considering research evidence, you need to think about how the work was carried out, and on whom, when and why. How was information analysed and presented? Do you feel the work presents relevant and useful information for you to use in caring for your patients? If not, what are the alternatives?

Of course, you are not expected to do this all on your own. Many books and journals offer advice on the critical review of papers; indeed, most healthcare research texts will demonstrate examples of tools that may be used.

Activity 1.11   *Reflection*

Now you have read this chapter, reflect on all the places you have seen nurses at work. Jot down the different workplaces and then try to identify how their jobs might be different.

- What nursing job would you do when you qualify?
- Why do you think this would be a good job to do?

Now look at the case studies in the summary document *Modernising Nursing Careers: Setting the direction* (DH, 2006).

- What do you think about these career trajectories?
- Are they the same as your ideas?
- Could you see yourself working in a different job when you qualify after reading these?

As this activity is based on your own reflection, there is no outline answer at the end of the chapter.

Chapter summary

Throughout this chapter, you have begun to explore the way that nursing is defined, and it is extremely complex. Many contextual influences, including geography and history, sociological concerns and professional ones, influence nursing. Nursing is also defined by the nature of the skills required to undertake it, how it is regulated and by national and international law. As you have seen, nursing is also not really identifiable as a single profession with the same activities for all; there are different types of nurses doing different types of work. It may be easier to define nursing as a family of different roles and activities. This is excellent news for the new nurse, because it offers wide and varied career pathways and many opportunities for development. A nursing career will not be the same every day, nor the same job over a number of years. When you talk to nurses about their career paths, you find that these are very individual. Nursing is a global career and some people move around, while others stay in the same place and change the types of jobs they might do. Nurses can be found in hospitals and clinics, in acute care settings and in long-term care settings. Nurses become managers, educators, researchers and even consultants.

Within this chapter, the definition of nursing focused on exploring external contextual influences relating to the work of nursing within society. However, this is not the whole story. In the next chapter you will explore a very different perspective on the definition of nursing. Chapter 2 focuses on the role of individual values and on the values of others. It considers how nursing is influenced by image and media in contemporary society and how nurses, are defined by their professional status. As you enter the profession of nursing, you will also be defined by these values.

Activities: brief outline answers

Activity 1.5 (page 13)

The Reporting of Injuries, Diseases and Dangerous Occurrence Regulations (RIDDOR) (HSE, 1995) apply to all workplaces and not just to nursing. However, they define the way that a nurse can work by virtue of the fact that the nurse has a responsibility to complete contemporaneous records of incidents. Some situations will be defined by local workplace policy and so untoward incidents must be reported to senior personnel. Some situations must be reported to the HSE.

Activity 1.9 (page 21)

These kinds of questions are important for consideration when planning care for a child like Jason.

- Admission to hospital may be the result of an infection in the first place and there is likely to be a need to manage this.
- Jason will need to be cared for in isolation, away from other children with infections, and this may be difficult for him and his family.
- The nurse will need to explain carefully to the family how to protect Jason, and may need to nurse him using special precautions to keep his environment clean.
- When Jason returns home there will be a need to balance Jason's emotional and social needs with his needs to be protected from infection.
- Nurses can help Jason's family to understand how to advise relatives and friends about visiting only when well themselves, and about how to maintain a clean environment for Jason.
- Jason's family will need lots of support and the nurse can help with this too.
- Counselling and resources are likely to be needed to both adapt the care environments and ensure provision of future support, as well as to advise on the genetic impact of the diagnosis.

It is fair to say that Jason's situation is a complex one for all concerned, and the outline answer to this activity offers only the smallest consideration of the many issues that may need to be addressed. But it does demonstrate the role of the nurse as both an advocate and a health promoter in enabling the best environment for care. For further information, visit **www.pia.org.uk/** and **www.ich.ucl.ac.uk/fact sheets/families/F040279/index.htmlx.htm**.

Further reading

Goodman, B and Clemow, R (2010) *Nursing and Collaborative Practice: A guide to interprofessional and interpersonal working*, 2nd edition. Exeter: Learning Matters.

A useful guide to interpersonal working relationships.

Mallik, M, Hall, C and Howard, D (2009) *Nursing Knowledge and Practice: Foundations for decision making*, 3rd edition. Edinburgh: Elsevier.

This is a text that advances thinking about the nursing introduced in this book. It considers knowledge for practice in greater depth and more specifically, and relates to the four fields of practice using a case study approach.

McHale, J and Tingle, J (2007) *Law and Nursing*, 3rd edition. Philadelphia: Butterworth-Heinemann-Elsevier.

This is a comprehensive consideration of the law and its impact on nursing. A useful reference text.

Royal College of Nursing (RCN) (2003) *Defining Nursing.* London: RCN.

This is a clearly written consideration of what makes nursing a unique profession. It is helpful for new nurses and also those who have been in the profession for a number of years.

Williamson, GR, Jenkinson, T and Proctor-Childs, T (2010) *Contexts of Contemporary Nursing,* 2nd edition. Exeter: Learning Matters.

A really useful introduction to the history of nursing as a profession within the wider healthcare system.

Useful websites

www.timelineindex.com/content/view/226

This website has a comprehensive timeline view of the development of mental healthcare in the UK.

Chapter 2
Being a professional nurse: image and values in nursing

Dawn Ritchie

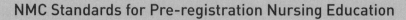

NMC Standards for Pre-registration Nursing Education

This chapter will address the following competencies:

Domain 1: Professional values

1. All nurses must practise with confidence according to *The Code: Standards of conduct, performance and ethics for nurses and midwives* (NMC 2008a), and within other recognised ethical and legal frameworks. They must be able to recognise and address ethical challenges relating to people's choices and decision making about their care, and act within the law to help them and their families and carers find acceptable solutions.
2. All nurses must practise in a holistic, non-judgmental, caring and sensitive manner that avoids assumptions, supports social inclusion; recognises and respects individual choice; and acknowledges diversity. Where necessary, they must challenge inequality, discrimination and exclusion from access to care.

Domain 2: Communication and interpersonal skills

5. All nurses must use therapeutic principles to engage, maintain and, where appropriate, disengage from professional caring relationships, and must always respect professional boundaries.

Domain 3: Nursing practice and decision making

6. All nurses must practise safely by being aware of the correct use, limitations and hazards of common interventions, including nursing activities, treatments, and the use of medical devices and equipment. The nurse must be able to evaluate their use, report any concerns promptly through appropriate channels and modify care where necessary to maintain safety. They must contribute to the collection of local and national data and formulation of policy on risks, hazards and adverse outcomes.

Domain 4: Leadership, management and team working

4. All nurses must be self-aware and recognise how their own values, principles and assumptions may affect their practice. They must maintain their own personal and professional development, learning from experience, through supervision, feedback, reflection and evaluation.

Introduction

In order to appreciate the diverse role of the nurse, this chapter will consider the key features of being a professional, which builds upon the exploration of nursing in Chapter 1. The development of a professional identity will be investigated by looking at how contemporary images and representations of nursing have evolved. You will also be challenged to explore further your own values and the value base within nursing, including how the value requirements for nurses are set down within the NMC *Code of Professional Conduct: Standards of conduct, performance and ethics* (*The Code*) (2008a). This will help to prepare you as a future nurse by gaining a better understanding of nurses and their responsibilities to patients and clients, carers and other healthcare professionals. The breadth of settings where nursing care is delivered, together with the changing role of the nurse within modern-day healthcare, is examined, including a discussion of the maintenance of a professional identity.

Nursing as a profession

Nursing has traditionally been regarded as a vocation, with nurses providing service to others. Vocation implies a divine calling, and is also possibly linked to the early roots of nursing within religious orders. The historical review provided an insight to how nursing has strived for professional status and, throughout the second half of the twentieth century, much was written about nursing being a profession. Not surprisingly, nurses tend to view themselves as professionals and want others to see them in the same light.

Activity 2.1 *Reflection*

*   What are the characteristics of a professional?
*   How do nurses become professional?

As this activity is based on your own reflection, there is no outline answer at the end of the chapter.

A profession is defined by the *Oxford English Dictionary* as *an occupation in which a professed knowledge of some subject, field, or science is applied; a vocation or career, especially one that involves prolonged training and a formal qualification.* Classically, the use of the term profession applied only to law, the Church (divinity) and medicine. Ideologically, the central features that define a profession include:

- altruistic service to society;
- developing and maintaining a distinct knowledge base – which may include a distinct vocabulary;
- autonomy – members of a profession are autonomous in practice, being able to make and act upon independent decisions;
- regulation or licensing of entrants to the profession following an education process;
- development of professional body;
- ethical codes and a culture of self-regulation.

In exploring definitions of a profession, it is vital that you consider your own perspectives, especially when one considers that not even all nurses agree that nursing is a profession.

When nursing is examined through traditional criteria of what constitutes a profession, it is apparent that some of the central features are missing or incomplete. In particular, nursing has difficulty in articulating a sufficient degree of nursing knowledge that is distinct from medicine. It is this discipline-specific knowledge that separates one profession from another. Historically, it can be argued that nursing derived knowledge from medicine, behavioural and social sciences. Nonetheless, it must also be recognised that, more recently, nursing has started to develop its own knowledge base, as demonstrated by the nursing models and frameworks of care discussed in Chapters 3 and 4.

Likewise, it can also be argued that another major professional characteristic that is missing from nursing is that of autonomy.

> *Nurses work in complex hierarchies where they are subordinate to organisational structures, professional agendas, and the culturally endorsed cognitive authority of medicine.*
> (Liaschenko and Peter, 2004, p489)

This does not mean that nurses are not able to make decisions about their clients; it means that the nature of contemporary nursing and the context in which care is delivered make it impossible for nurses to be self-sufficient in their decision making. Nursing is not unique in being in this position, since other public sector occupations, including teaching and social work, are also what Etzioni (1969) describes as semi-professions and the Office for National Statistics (ONS, 2000) UK Standard Occupational Classification System suggests are associate professional occupations. However, social and cultural changes over the last three decades, together with organisational changes in the delivery of health services, including the Wanless Report (2002), Knowledge and Skills Framework (KSF) (DH, 2004a) and Agenda for Change (DH, 2004b), have stimulated evaluation of professional roles and core values. Rather than debating whether nursing is a profession, vocation or occupation, the focus has shifted towards examination and redistribution of roles and exploration of the concept of professionalism.

Concept summary: Health Service initiatives

The Wanless Report

The Wanless Report (2002) was an evidence-based assessment of the long-term resource requirements for the NHS. It emphasised the need for reform and increased investment in order to improve public health and reduce health inequalities. Details are available at **www.hmtreasury.gov.uk/Consultations_and_Legislation/wanless/consult_wanless_final.cfm**.

The Knowledge and Skills Framework

The Knowledge and Skills Framework (KSF) is essentially about lifelong learning. It is a generic framework that defines and describes the knowledge and skills NHS staff require to carry out their work effectively and thereby move forward with the development of services to meet the needs of service users. It is intended to facilitate individual learning and development via a review process that promotes equality and diversity for all staff. Details are available at **www.dh.gov.uk/en/Publicationsandstatistics/Publications/CommunicationsSummary/index.htm**.

Agenda for Change

The KSF is one of the three strands within the NHS Agenda for Change. Agenda for Change is the name given to the new NHS pay and grading system implemented in 2004, which allows career progression based on the knowledge and skills applied to jobs. Details are available at **www.nhsemployers.org/pay-conditions/agenda-for-change.cfm**.

Being professional

Being professional suggests membership of a privileged occupational group and also possession of certain interpersonal attributes, including knowledge, skills and attitudes. The public generally accord nurses professional status, albeit with different meanings from the traditional notions, and by virtue of such have expectations of nurses as both individuals and collectively. In particular, the public have an expectation for nurses to be trustworthy and always to act in the best interests of their patients. Nursing, in common with other professions, has published statements about what qualified members are competent to do and what people can reasonably expect.

The initial period for developing proficiency and achieving the minimum occupational standards in nursing is the pre-registration training, when you will be helped to develop the knowledge and skills that will enable you to become a registered nurse. As a nursing student you are required to gain experience by undertaking a specified number of theoretical hours and completing practice experience in particular nursing practice placements. In the UK, entry to the profession was formalised with the passing of the Nurses Registration Act in 1919, when it became a statutory requirement to be registered in order to practise. The NMC maintains a register of practitioners who have met the standards for entry to the profession, currently 670,000 registrants (**www.nmc-uk.org**). This mechanism of statutory registration ensures that nurses have achieved the proficiencies described in statute. These are currently set out as NMC *Standards for Pre-registration Nursing Education* (2010) in accordance with the Nursing and Midwifery Order 2001 – Statutory Instrument 2004/254, and can also be accessed via the NMC website above. These standards are concerned with ensuring the protection of the public. The public quite rightly expects that a qualified nurse will be competent when carrying out the normal tasks and duties of a nurse. This is frequently referred to as a practitioner being fit to practise.

Four domains of practice have been identified as essential for registration purposes:

- professional values;
- communication and decision making;
- nursing practice and decision making;
- leadership, management and team working.

These domains are comprised of a generic standard for competence which all nurses must achieve and a field standard for competence which must be achieved by nurses in each specific field, i.e. adult nursing, mental health nursing, learning disabilities nursing and children's nursing. These are further broken down into clear statements of what is to be learned during your pre-registration training, competencies. Throughout the practice component of your nurse training you will be continuously assessed against these criteria. A nurse mentor who has completed specific preparation in assessing students is normally responsible for assessment in practice settings. These competencies are the same for all pre-registration courses, whatever academic level you are studying at, e.g., degree, masters, or postgraduate level. Progression towards professional qualification occurs generally at the end of each year, separating the programme into three equal parts. Successful completion of each part is required prior to advancing into the next part. Before you can apply to the NMC for professional registration you must have acquired all the generic and field competency requirements in each domain for your specific field of practice, that is, adult, mental health, learning disability or child nursing.

Activity 2.2   *Research and reflection*

Look up the websites for the NMC (**www.nmc-uk.org**) and the Council for Healthcare Regulatory Excellence (CHRE – **www.chre.org.uk**). In the light of what you find there, consider whether the regulation of healthcare professionals is necessary.

Why might this be?

Does regulation automatically confer professional status?

Outline answers are given at the end of the chapter.

Learning and development of proficiency continue well beyond registration and there is an obligation within both the NMC *Code* (2008a) and within the NHS KSF for all registered nurses to engage in continuing professional development (CPD). Throughout a professional career, individual scope of competence will change as a consequence of an expanding knowledge base that leads to increasing specialism. In addition, the increasing complexity of healthcare has meant that nurses have moved, and will continue to move, into developing areas of practice.

As well as possessing knowledge and skills, professionalism is demonstrated by our attitudes and behaviours, qualities that characterise a profession. Qualities considered necessary for nurses to possess include honesty, integrity, compassion, altruism, listening skills, excellence and multi-disciplinary working. As part of *Nursing Standard*'s 2005 *Nursing the Future* campaign, nursing's core values were defined as follows.

- **Compassion** – means to suffer and includes the desire to relieve the distress or suffering of another.
- **Teamwork** – a fundamental feature of modern healthcare requiring knowledge and understanding of other disciplines.
- **Make a difference** – is possibly the value that, as individuals, we find most difficult to define. As a profession we continue to debate and are unable to define precisely what constitutes nursing knowledge and skills. However, caring is frequently what the public tell us makes a difference.
- **Versatility** – critical to versatility is being able to demonstrate competence and knowledge of nursing. As nurses we need to be able to learn broadly as well as focusing on our specific field areas.

The large circled values in Figure 2.1 represent planets or the core fixed values of nursing. Circling around them, the smaller circles represent moons or the secondary characteristics of nursing. These are acknowledged as being diverse and changeable, and can even be contradictory.

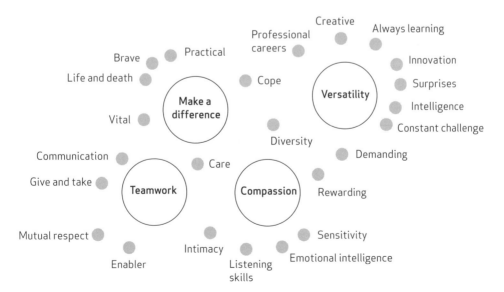

Figure 2.1: The desired core values of nursing.

Source: The desired core values of nursing: analysis diagram of the *Nursing Standard* Magazine Workshop. November 2004. *Nursing Standard*, 19(30), 6 April 2005.

These values are also reflected within the NMC's *Code*, which requires you to:

- *make the care of people your first concern, treating them as individuals and respecting their dignity;*
- *work with others to protect and promote the health and wellbeing of those in your care, their families and carers, and the wider community;*
- *provide a high standard of practice and care at all times;*
- *be open and honest, act with integrity and uphold the reputation of your profession.*

(NMC, 2008a)

Activity 2.3   *Reflection*

As a profession, consideration needs to be given as to what nursing's core values are. A value can be defined as being the ideas that we believe are important, and the things that we regard and rank highly. They can be owned either by an individual or by a group as a whole.

What are your core values?

Can you identify a time when your personal values may come into conflict with the requirement to uphold the NMC *Code*?

As this activity is based on your own reflection, there is no outline answer at the end of the chapter.

Professionalism and the student nurse

Eraut (1994) suggests that a professional person's competence has two dimensions: scope and quality. Scope refers to the range of tasks, roles and situations for which competence is determined, whereas quality pertains to judgement about the standard of work. The standard of work takes into account the level at which the individual is working and, as already discussed, is defined by the NMC. Level of competence will vary depending upon whether it is a novice who is not yet proficient in a task or someone who is regarded as being an expert. As a student nurse you are required to work under the direct supervision of a registered nurse. Initially, this will mean that you are always accompanied by your mentor, but as your knowledge, skills, experience and confidence develop you will find yourself in situations where you are not directly accompanied. As a student it is imperative that you do not participate in any activity for which you have not been fully prepared or where you are not adequately supervised, since it is expected that you should recognise the limitations of your own abilities. Should you encounter a situation that you perceive as beyond your abilities and for which you have not been adequately prepared or supervised, you must refer back to a registered nurse. If you choose to undertake an activity that is beyond your capabilities, you can be called to account for your actions or omissions either by your university and/or by the law.

Inexperience is not a defence, since you would be reasonably expected to recognise that you could not carry out the task. As highlighted in Chapter 1, although you are never professionally accountable in the way you would be following registration, that is, you cannot be called to account by the NMC, you can still be called to account by your university or by the law. It is therefore apparent that student nurses do have accountability to their level of training and to their expertise, and they do have an ethical duty to promote and protect the well-being of patients.

The law primarily exists to deter bad behaviour. While every registered nurse has a legal duty of care to do the patient no harm, there is also an ethical duty of care that requires the nurse to promote the well-being of the patient. This is encapsulated within the NMC *Code* (2007a). It could therefore be postulated that the ethical duty of care is more stringent than the legal duty of care. All student nurses have an ethical duty of care by virtue of their special relationship and direct contact with patients. Because of this the patient has certain rights and the nurse has certain obligations, such as respecting the wishes of patients at all times, maintaining confidentiality and acting fairly and sensitively. As a student you do need to recognise professional biases and base actions and decisions upon sound rationale. It must be remembered that the patient always comes first. Patients have the right to refuse to allow students to participate in caring for them and consent must be sought from the patient. The needs and rights of the patient will always supersede the needs of the student.

Concept summary: Ethical principles

Beauchamp and Childress (1994) identified the four ethical principles underpinning healthcare practice as:

- *respect for autonomy* – respecting people's wishes to be self-determined, their dignity and decisions; promoting well-being; and treating people with honesty and truthfulness;
- *beneficence* – promoting well-being and doing good;
- *non-maleficence* – doing no harm, weighing up the benefits and burdens of any actions; although we have an ethical duty to promote the well-being of patients, this does have be tempered against the right of the individual to refuse treatment and consideration of whether the treatment is an excessive burden;
- *justice* – treating all individuals fairly and equitably, not discriminating on the grounds of race, gender, religion, etc. We also need to consider the resource implications and finite nature of healthcare.

Student behaviour is not just about competence to perform a skill; it is also about demonstrating personal integrity and fitness for practice. Examples of professional integrity include being able to be trusted with the property of others, being able to be trusted with confidential information, accurate completion of care delivery records, showing compassion for others and responding appropriately to the emotional needs of patients and their families, and demonstrating respect for individuals. (This is not an exhaustive list.) The personal integrity of anyone in contact with vulnerable clients is paramount. This helps to explain why both admission to a nursing programme and entrance to the NMC register is a rigorous process. The NMC requires universities to ensure that processes are in place to assess and ensure that students are in good health and of good character at admission to, during and on completion of pre-registration nursing programmes. It is essential that you remember that registration is not simply an administrative procedure. It is only when you have met the required standards and the pre-registration course director completes a declaration of good health and character on your behalf that you will be eligible for entry on to the NMC register.

Good health means that you must be able to undertake safe and effective practice as a registered nurse without supervision (NMC, 2008a). It does not mean that you cannot be a nurse should you suffer from a disability or chronic illness, provided that the health problem doesn't render you unfit to be safe and effective in carrying out your duties. There is an obligation upon employers through the Equality Act (2010) which applies in England, Scotland and Wales to make reasonable adjustments. An impairment or health condition is considered on an individual basis. The act does not apply in Northern Ireland where the Disability Discrimination Act 1995, the Disability Discrimination Act 2005 which amended the Disability Discrimination Act 1995, and the Disability Discrimination (Northern Ireland) Order 2006 apply. Further clarification can be found on the Equality and Human Rights Commission website at **www.equalityhuman rights.com**.

Similarly, should you have a temporary health problem, this would not mean that you are not fit to practise, since you should make a full recovery and be able to return to finish your pre-registration programme.

Nurses are required by the public and profession to be honest and trustworthy. The NMC (**www.nmc-uk.org**) states that:

> *Good character is important and is central to the code in that nurses must be honest and trustworthy. Good character is based on an individual's conduct, behaviour and attitude. It also takes account of any convictions, cautions and pending charges that are likely to be incompatible with professional registration. A person's character must be sufficiently good for them to be capable of safe and effective practice without supervision.*

Activity 2.4   *Critical thinking*

Consider the following situations. You may find it beneficial to look at the NMC website, at the *Guidance on Professional Conduct for Nursing and Midwifery Students* (2010) (**www.nmc-uk.org/Students/Guidance-for-students/**).

1. Two students conduct a discussion on Facebook about their activities while on a learning experience and also include some explicit photographs of their recent night out.
   - What are the professional implications of using social networking sites?
2. A student has had 46 days of sickness during the first year of the nursing preparation programme. The student has not attended theory and practice sessions but has provided no medical evidence to support ill-health claims either.

continued opposite . . .

continued . . .

- What are the professional implications of this behaviour?
- If the student has lied about illness, what does this say about the individual's honesty and personal integrity?

3. A student nurse is celebrating New Year's Eve until the early hours of the morning and consumes an excessive amount of alcohol. The student is on an early shift on New Year's Day and, while driving to learning experience, is stopped by the police and breathalysed. The student is found to be over the legal drink–drive alcohol limit.

   - What is the student's obligation to the university and what are the implications of this action for the student?

Outline answers are provided at the end of the chapter.

Images of nursing

In order to explore further the professional role of the nurse, it is useful to consider the way in which the image of both nurses and nursing as a profession has evolved.

Healthcare is rarely out of the media spotlight, whether it is about innovations in treatment and care, or about the 'usual' falling apart and imminent demise of the NHS. The state of the NHS remains one of the most important and contentious issues facing politicians. The media has tremendous power in its ability to affect the public's perceptions of healthcare and yet, within these stories, nurses continue to be perceived by the public in a predominantly stereotypical manner. As Berry (2004) acknowledged, a profession's media image is an indicator of its political, social and economic value, which may in turn impact upon the allocation of resources, recruitment and retention of staff, and in addition influence morale within the profession.

Nursing is a caring profession and the challenge for nurses is to personify the public's image of the caring professional nurse. As highlighted earlier, professionalism relates to a set of values, behaviours and relationships that are integral to the regulation of the profession and underpin the trust the public places in nurses. It has already been identified that the desired professional image for nurses is to be described as being competent, trustworthy and caring; however, in the increasingly diverse twenty-first century, nurses face a number of complex challenges in maintaining a positive professional image. A dichotomy frequently exists between how nursing is envisioned and what actually occurs. Although it can be argued that the image of the nursing profession as a whole has become somewhat devalued over the last few decades, people don't tend to regard their 'own nurse' to be like that and in general there is a high regard for individual nurses.

A stereotype is a generalisation about a person or group of people, which does not acknowledge individual differences and which is often prejudicial to that person or group. Society often innocently creates and perpetuates stereotypes, but these stereotypes can be harmful since they are not necessarily valid or accurate and can lead, on occasion, to discrimination and harassment.

Commonly, people will form an opinion about another individual based on their appearance, posture or language.

Activity 2.5   *Reflection*

From what you already know, reflect on stereotypes of nurses.

- What are they linked to? Where do they originate from?
- Have they changed over the years?
- Do they vary according to the field of nursing (i.e. adult, child, learning disability or mental health)?
- Do they vary according to nationality/cultural grouping?

As this activity is based on your own reflection, and the answers are discussed in the text, there is no outline answer at the end of the chapter.

Nursing has for many years been represented within the media as being a feminine occupation (Hallam, 1998). Likewise, a common perception of British people is that they are shy and reserved with their emotions. These generalisations have their origins in what individuals may have been told by family and friends, what they may have experienced themselves, what they may have read in books and magazines, and what they may have seen on television and in films. The problem with these generalisations is that what may be true of the group as a whole may not apply to individuals within that group.

The stereotyping of nursing has historically paralleled the portrayal of women within society (Hallam, 1998). Bridges (1990) identified 34 different types of stereotypes associated with nurses. Darbyshire (2002) suggested that it could be considered 'a back-handed compliment' that so many stereotypes are associated with nursing. Nevertheless, nurses' perception of how others view them has been demonstrated by Takase et al. (2002) to impact not only on the development of individual confidence and collective self-esteem, but also on job satisfaction. Stereotypes can have both positive and negative connotations. The difficulty of positive stereotypes is whether you can ever live up to expectations. Equally, it may not be possible to overcome the damaging attributes that are associated with more negative stereotypes.

Stereotypes of nurses

The word 'nurse' is derived from the Latin *nutrire*, meaning to nourish or suckle, and the original meaning was of one who suckles a child who is not her own. The term nurse was therefore historically considered to embody the feminine attributes of tenderness, sensitivity and nurturing. Bridges (1990) identifies the four stereotypes that are the most recognisable to the wider public:

- ministering angel;
- battle-axe;
- naughty nurse;
- doctor's handmaiden.

The ministering angel

Perhaps the most enduring of all the stereotypes is that of the nurse as an 'angel'. Some of the earliest representations of nursing are based on nursing's origins within the religious orders. Nursing was viewed as a sacred service founded, according to Hallett (2007), on the concept of 'caritas', meaning charity, and encompassing the qualities of altruism and self-sacrifice. Prior to the 1800s, the sick were often looked after in workhouses or within the home by women of low repute, as portrayed by Sairey Gamp in Charles Dickens' nineteenth-century novel, *Martin Chuzzlewit*. However, it was Florence Nightingale who led the transformation of nurses from disreputable, drunken and debauched members of society, to the widely accepted stereotype of the nurse as the ministering angel. Nightingale's influence on promoting a positive image of nursing is indisputable and possibly reflects the cultural shift in Victorian times, when nursing became an acceptable occupation for young women, as opposed to being work solely for the socially undesirable. More recently, during the early part of the twentieth century, as Kallisch and Kallisch (1983) brought to attention, cinema portrayals of Florence Nightingale in films, such as *The White Angel* (1936) and *The Lady with the Lamp* (1951), romanticised and perpetuated the angelic image of nursing. This angelic image has generated societal expectations of nurses to be selfless, devoted, above reproach and saintly, and is one that still today pervades the media, being a recurrent theme within headlines.

Then again, together with the positive allusion of nurses as angels come the more negative connotations. The notion of vocation and self-sacrifice implicit within the stereotype of the angel image has, according to Cunningham (1999), perpetuated the notion that remuneration for the job is immaterial. This lack of remuneration can be traced back to Victorian times, and Bradley (1999, p16) describes the two types of Victorian nursing students: *ordinary probationers who were paid a small salary and the lady probationers who were paid board and lodging but received no remuneration.* Cunningham goes as far as to suggest that any perceived suffering of nurses only heightens their righteousness and morality. Yet this acceptance of low pay did have, and continues to have, repercussions upon the recruitment and retention of staff.

Perhaps more significantly, nurses are human and unable consistently to attain the perfection demanded by their angelic image, and this has been reflected in recent media portrayals. Critical documentaries, including the BBC *Panorama* programme, *Undercover Nurse* (2005), and the Channel 4 documentary, *Undercover Angels* (2005), have highlighted images of nurses as being uncaring, disrespectful and on occasions neglectful in their care. This has also been replicated within UK press when the media, particularly during August 2009, utilised angelic imagery when nurses' behaviour and role were brought into question. The difficulty appears to be in being able to overcome the traditional angelic imagery and portray nurses as skilled professionals who, while valuing care and compassion, are able to think critically and act independently. The saintly image of nurses has been eroded and, even if the myth has not yet been dispelled, the halo has most definitely slipped.

The battle-axe

The stereotypical image of the battle-axe is that of a matriarchal older female, who is extremely large, sexually unattractive and frequently bullying in nature. The battle-axe has been characterised by Nurse Ratched in the film, *One Flew Over the Cuckoo's Nest* (1975), and Annie Wilkes in Steven King's *Misery* (1990). The battle-axe has also been portrayed as a comic figure, the most well-known portrayal being that of Hattie Jacques as the Matron in the *Carry On* film series. This image of the matron arose following the end of the Second World War, at a time when society was having to adjust to the changing role of women and the growing influence of film and television. It is a stereotype that has endured over time and, recently, the government has responded to the general public's demand to bring back the authoritarian figure with the introduction of modern matrons. To a certain extent, the government has recently attempted to perpetuate and reinvent the battle-axe image with matrons being portrayed as 'taking charge' of wards, being responsible for the actions of staff and carrying out affirmative action when necessary to protect the interests of patients.

The naughty nurse

The naughty nurse stereotype is both reinforced and reflected by the media and relates to the intimate nature of caring for patients. As Darbyshire states, *having seen and touched the bodies of strangers, nurses are perceived as willing and able sexual partners* (2002, p41). This stereotype also reinforces the correlation between nursing and female gender stereotypes (Jinks and Bradley, 2004). It is interesting to note that the sexual objectification of nursing became dominant during the 1960s and 1970s. At this time, the modern feminist movement, which was committed to securing and defending women's rights and ensuring equal opportunities, was at its most prominent. Despite the constantly evolving role of women within society, sexual connotations continue to be perpetuated in the media, although Payne (2000) suggests that there is some evidence that the public are no longer influenced by this image.

The doctor's handmaiden

The image of the nurse as the doctor's handmaiden emerged in the nineteenth century, when nursing was seen as subordinate to the medical profession. It is possibly a relic of nurses' links to domestic workers and the so-called 'militarisation' of nursing that occurred following the Crimean, and the First and Second World Wars. Hallett (2007) suggests that, following this period, nursing *developed a rigid and routinised ethos* (p429). The power relation between doctors and nurses is clearly evident with the nurses' role being determined by the delegation of tasks from the doctor and an expectation that these would be followed without question.

Activity 2.6   *Reflection*

To what extent do stereotypical representations of nursing correspond to your own?

- Are the images positive? negative? neutral?
- To what extent do the representations link to reality?
- Are they linked to personal or second-hand experience?

As this activity is based on your own reflection, there is no outline answer at the end of the chapter.

The gap between the image of nursing in popular culture and the actual role that nurses undertake is growing. Although there is a multitude of factors as to why this may be so, the main reason for this disparity continues to be the fact that nursing is enduringly a female-dominated profession.

Nurses do appear to be mostly depicted in a negative manner, particularly by the media. Within the medium of television, nurses are still portrayed as doctors' handmaidens, who are unskilled and there to clean up after medical staff, that is, when they are not tending to doctors' hearts. For example, in a recent episode of the American drama *House*, the lead character, Dr Gregory House (played by Hugh Laurie), suggested that he considers nurses as being good only for handling stool specimens and assisting patients who have fallen down. Thus, the public perception that nurses are not competent and knowledgeable professionals, unlike medical staff, is perpetuated. Likewise, British television programmes such as Channel 4's *No Angels* keep alive the image of nurses as sex objects, but it could be postulated that programmes such as the BBC series *Casualty* and *Holby City* have attempted to portray nurses and nursing in a more realistic manner. However, these two programmes continue to promote the illusion that all nursing takes place within an acute hospital setting and do not portray the diversity of environments within which contemporary nursing care is delivered. For example, care delivery is increasingly occurring within a community setting. Since the media has an immeasurable power to influence, educate and enlighten the public, it is essential that nurses' roles are accurately represented.

Activity 2.7   *Critical thinking*

Read Jinks and Bradley (2004) Angel, handmaiden, battleaxe or whore? A study which examines changes in newly recruited student nurses' attitudes to gender and nursing stereotypes. *Nurse Education Today*, 24(2): 121–7.

- Why do you think that there has been a change between the 1992 and 2002 beliefs in gender and nursing stereotypes?
- Why does the handmaiden stereotype remain so enduring?

Now read Spouse (2000) 'An impossible dream? Images of nursing held by preregistration students and their effect on sustaining motivation to become nurses'. *Journal of Advanced Nursing*, 32(3): 730–9.

continued overleaf . . .

continued . . .

- Reflect upon what your image and understanding of nursing was prior to commencing training and following practice learning experiences. How have your beliefs, attitudes and values been challenged? Define for yourself what makes a 'good' or 'bad' nurse.
- How do your image and behaviour impact on both your patients and also the general public's perception of you as an individual and also as a professional?

As this activity is based on your own reflection and observations, there is no outline answer at the end of the chapter.

The demographics of undergraduate nursing students in the UK have changed dramatically over the last century and yet, as Fletcher (2007) identified, nurses are portrayed in the media as female, single, childless, white and under 35 years of age. So what does this mean for nursing students who are not from the majority group?

Increasingly, mature students who have a range of demanding responsibilities including juggling family life with a return to study, are deciding to undertake nurse training. Such mature students are expected to be able to both relate to students who may be of a much younger generation and fit in with them. Members of academic and clinical staff may be under the common mis-conception that, because of their maturity and life experiences, mature students are somehow better able to cope and adapt. However, Kevern and Webb (2004) identified that mature students often lack coping strategies and support systems. Challenges include having to adapt to playing the role of the student again, in addition to coping with changes in educational delivery and even technology. Relationships with supervisors in the academic setting and mentors in the clinical setting can be difficult, as some students may find it hard to accept guidance from younger mentors and supervisors. Unconsciously, they may feel that they should have certain knowledge. Developing an adult-to-adult relationship can be emotionally challenging and takes perseverance.

Numbers of male students within nursing have been increasing: the proportion of male registrants on the NMC register broke the 10 per cent barrier in 2002 and continues on a long-term upward trend, being recorded at 10.73 per cent in 2006. In many situations, gender is irrelevant and there are some individuals who particularly enjoy being in a minority. Many male students will be supervised by females and in the majority of cases this works well, but there are times when a male student may encounter difficulties as a result of not having a male role model. It can result in difficulties in developing an appropriate self-image and on occasions it may allow prejudices to manifest themselves, including exclusion and isolation. There may also be problems with males having to avoid sexual innuendo. One of the implications surrounding male nurses is that they have traditionally been perceived as being effeminate, as real men don't undertake care. Likewise, there is also a perception that male nurses will be attracted to the more technological aspects of care or management (Macintosh, 1997). There is a need for research into the image and reality of men in nursing. The effects of such stereotyping are considerable and may result in a great deal of stress. When people make remarks and comments about a stereotype and then imply that something is wrong or abnormal, it can lead to individuals being a target for dis-crimination and harassment. This can cause considerable distress and interfere with an individual's ability to work. Harassment and discrimination are offences and legal sanctions can be used against perpetrators.

Activity 2.8   *Reflection*

Reflect on your experiences of the four fields of pre-registration nursing and think about any images that you may have associated with each fields of nursing. Now consider to what extent these images have influenced your beliefs and attitudes. Following exposure to the different fields of nursing, have your attitudes changed?

As this activity is based on your own reflection and observations, there is no outline answer at the end of the chapter.

So why is image important?

As individuals, we define ourselves and are defined by others through images. Our image defines the way we behave, the way others respond and behave towards us and our confidence in our own self. Nursing too is defined by image. Image is of importance since it reflects societal values of nurses and the nursing profession (Hallam, 1998). The way in which the public perceives nursing significantly influences nurses' job satisfaction.

The NMC set out standards for conduct, performance and ethics for nursing and midwifery professions within the *Code of Professional Conduct* (NMC, 2008a), which informs the public, other professions and employers of the standard of professional conduct they can expect in a registered practitioner.

As a registered nurse, midwife or specialist community public health nurse, you are personally accountable for your practice. In caring for patients and clients, you must:

- *respect the patient or client as an individual;*
- *obtain consent before you give any treatment or care;*
- *protect confidential information;*
- *cooperate with others in the team;*
- *maintain your professional knowledge and competence;*
- *be trustworthy;*
- *act to identify and minimise risk to patients and clients.*

These are the shared values of all the United Kingdom healthcare regulatory bodies.

| Activity 2.9 | *Research and critical thinking* |

Obtain a copy of the NMC *Code of Professional Conduct: Standards for conduct, performance and ethics*, which can be found on the NMC website (**www.nmc-uk.org**) under publications.

Discuss with another student, or in small groups, the professional behaviour expected of registered nurses. Consider why different standards of behaviour may be expected of you as a student nurse studying for both a professional and academic award, from standards expected of other students who are studying for an award that is academic only.

Consider other healthcare professionals, such as social workers, occupational therapists, physiotherapists and doctors. What values and codes of conduct inform their practice? In what ways are these similar or different?

Check the websites of the following organisations:

- General Social Care Council (**www.gscc.org.uk**);
- Chartered Society of Physiotherapy (**www.csp.org.uk**);
- British Association of Occupational Therapists (**www.cot.org.uk**);
- Health Professions Council (**www.hpc-uk.org**);
- General Medical Council (**www.gmc.org.uk**).

Identify some of the common concerns that may bring into question a student's fitness to practise.

Outline answers are provided at the end of the chapter.

Professional image incorporates a number of facets and is about how nurses present themselves in public and in private settings. Knowingly or unknowingly, appearance, interactions and communication with others, behaviour and the people with whom nurses associate are all components of the image projected to the general public and are, therefore, part of the defining image of nursing.

The importance of appearance in creating a positive and professional image cannot be overstated. Appearance can engender and enhance the confidence of patients and clients, their families and colleagues by giving the impression of professional competence. However, a professional identity and image is not only defined by the way we dress, but also by the way we communicate and behave. Nurses are required to build relationships with patients and clients, their families, colleagues and other professionals based on honesty, openness, trust, respect and good communication.

As nurses, it is important to recognise that all patients and clients are individuals who can expect to be addressed in a professional manner, as you would expect to both address, and be addressed by, other professionals. The nursing profession is made up of individual people and, as identified by Fletcher (2007), the public develop their construction and perception of the profession through these individuals.

Activity 2.10   *Research and critical thinking*

Think about how you introduce yourself to patients and clients.

- Do you use your first name? last name? your title?
- If you are not fully introducing yourself, what are the implications for the individual you are caring for?
- How does this impact upon the public's perception of nursing?

As this activity is based on your own reflection, and the answers are discussed in the text, there is no outline answer at the end of the chapter.

A large proportion of nurses identify themselves without using their last names or titles. The Kennedy Report of the Bristol Royal Infirmary Inquiry (Kennedy, 2001) acknowledged that nurses frequently reverse their identity badges, or cover their last names so that they cannot be recognised. In paediatric areas it is not uncommon for staff to decorate their badges with stickers so that nobody can possibly read their name. This means that the nurse is unable to be identified as an individual and this is contrary to the patient's right to know the full name, title and function of the person caring for them.

Nursing as a graduate profession

In the UK, tremendous debate has taken place for several decades as to whether nursing should be an all-graduate profession. The Department of Health announced in 2009 that, following a review of standards of pre-registration nurse education in the UK, all new nurses will have to be educated to degree level from September 2013. Becoming an all-graduate profession is, according to Bernhauser (2010), core to meeting the challenges of delivering healthcare in the twenty-first century. Graduate entry registration is in the nurse's best interests, the interests of the profession and also in the interests of the patients for whom they care.

Pre-registration nurse education in England is arguably the last major profession to make the transition to degree-level qualification – midwifery and allied health professions have already made this shift. Requiring degree level education and preparation as a minimum will not only help to create a stronger professional identity, but also reduce educational disparity with other members of the health and social care team. Considerable differences of opinion exist in relation to this move with the time-honoured image of the nurse facing erosion. Interestingly, no concerns were raised when midwifery and other professions allied to health became all graduate, and perhaps much of the debate relates to the myths and misperceptions between image and the reality of nursing. The traditional apprenticeship style of nurse training, where students acquired skills and knowledge 'on the job', is often espoused as having provided nurses with the best education. It is counter-productive to think that graduate nurses will be able to 'hit the ground running' at the point of registration in the same way. In order to support transition to being a member of the workforce, preceptorship/mentoring schemes are essential for newly qualified nurses (discussed in Chapter 6). It must also be remembered that the traditional apprenticeship style of training, where students were employees, enabled the needs of service to take precedence but failed to provide for the learning needs of students, which was demonstrated by high levels of attrition. It has also been recognised as having failed to equip nurses with the skills required to respond to both changing healthcare needs and advances in care delivery with Greenwood (2000) suggesting that it generated nurses who were 'doers rather than thinkers'.

There are general public concerns about the move to an all-graduate profession in particular around safety, quality and the notion that 'education' and 'caring' are mutually exclusive. Nurses do need to work hard to retain public respect and confidence. There exists a tacit assumption that an educated nurse will not be either a caring or a competent nurse despite there being no evidence existing to support this. As Watson (2000) declared, 'there has never been a concomitant suggestion that Doctors are too well educated'. Currently, there is minimal public awareness that pre-registration nursing students have been gaining their education in universities, with increasing numbers being educated to degree and masters level. The establishment of graduate nurses has been occurring over the last few decades within the UK, and although this has been a slow-moving process it is estimated that just over a quarter of registered nurses in England hold a qualification at degree level or above. Scotland and Wales have already moved to only offering degree-level pre-registration nursing programmes, and Northern Ireland will follow to an all degree programme from 2011. The change to degree-level registration will bring all UK nurse education up to the same level as that in the majority of Europe, Australia, New Zealand and the USA.

Caution needs to be applied when extrapolating from existing research. However, studies do provide a number of insights as to the possible benefits of an all-graduate profession, which include the following.

- Equipping nurses to be critical thinkers who question practice, and demonstrate effective clinical decision-making skills.
- Improved patient outcomes with Aiken (2003) suggesting that better educated nurses deliver higher quality care.
- Enhanced expertise with graduates possessing a broader range of technical, analytical, managerial and leadership skills.
- Contrary to a widely held myth, Watson (2000) indicates that graduate nurses remain in clinical practice longer and have better decision-making skills. US studies also indicate that they are less likely to leave the profession.
- Parity with other professions, a degree being a universal currency for employers and also seen to be essential for career progression.
- Evidence has shown that for other professions, such as teaching, when the entry level was increased the popularity of the profession improved.

Nursing in the UK is currently in a transition phase, and is liable to remain so for a number of years. There is a requirement to ensure that the integration of an all-graduate profession is well thought out and efficiently implemented. During this phase we do need to ensure that a wide entry gate to the profession remains since although there is evidence that some candidates will be encouraged to apply for degree-level study, others such as mature students are likely to be deterred. Robinson and Bennett (2007) suggest that there is mixed evidence on the effects of graduate status on diversity. Consideration must be made to prior education and experience, learning pathways and appropriate student support during pre-registration period.

A simultaneous commitment to existing registered nurses is essential to ensure that they feel highly valued since the impact on the existing workforce is likely to be great. Even within the current climate of cost containment, there must be continuing professional development opportunities, including the opportunity to advance to degree level. It is also incumbent on both academic and service colleagues to develop strategies to support the existing nursing workforce with graduate transition since mentoring students in the practice setting plays a vital role in shaping students' values, attitudes and behaviours. MacLeod Clark (2008) suggests that the nursing profession must positively embrace this transformation and acknowledge that it is likely the shape of the profession will change and there will be fewer registered nurses. Developing roles at assistant practitioner level is likely to be essential in terms of both recruiting students and in maintaining a wide entry gate to an all-graduate pre-registration programme. Since the educational standard was raised in Australia and New Zealand, those countries have become increasingly dependent on second-level nurses. Professional boundaries have become less clear over time with the blurring of roles between doctors, allied healthcare professionals, registered nurses and support workers. This role redesign is vital to the implementation of the *NHS Plan* (DH, 2000) and National Service Frameworks (NSFs) and is also reflected within the aims of *Liberating the Talents* (DH, 2002) and *New Ways of Working* (NHS Modernisation Agency, 2003). By breaking down interprofessional boundaries, it allows health service managers far greater flexibility in the deployment of staff.

Nurses are the largest single profession within the Health Service and the nursing profession has recently received unprecedented scrutiny as a consequence of controversies, changing working practices and increased public expectations. The public expect nurses to be competent, compassionate, and caring. Fradd (2010) claims that patients want nurses who can:

- communicate well;
- be organised;
- be confident;
- be competent;
- practise safely;
- navigate them through complicated services;
- maintain good relationships;
- construct rational arguments on their behalf;
- enable them to make informed decisions.

Bringing in degree-level registration is intended to ensure that nurses are better equipped to meet the challenges of the increased complexity of patient care and the changing needs of consumers to benefit the delivery of contemporary healthcare.

Degree-level study

Students arriving at university frequently comment on how degree-level study is different from anything they have done before. Students often want to continue in the same style of learning that they have experienced at school and college. They can find the challenge of independent learning demanding as they may not have fully developed skills in time management and self-direction, which can then impact on their motivation to learn. University students will not be chased up by their lecturers to see if they have completed work. Likewise, more mature students may find limitations in direct contact time frustrating, especially when they may perceive that they have made personal and financial sacrifices to undertake the programme. Pre-registration nursing students are unlike traditional university students since they are not only studying for an academic award but are also studying for professional registration, which can result in a failure to appreciate just how much work is required. When they start practice placements, students will be required to work unsocial hours, including early shifts, late shifts, long days (usually 12-hour shifts), night shifts and weekends. This can be very testing when peers undertaking more traditional academic programmes may only have as little as six hours taught time/direct contact time per week. Progression points usually occur at the end of each academic year and nursing students must not only meet the university requirements for academic progression but also practice requirements. Usually, the academic results obtained during Year One do not count towards the final degree classification and a number of students do readily admit that they could have put more effort into their first-year assessments. Likewise, the transition to degree-level study in Year 3 can be as difficult as the initial transition to university. Both the academic and practice requirements are greatly increased in terms of competence, critical thinking, reflection and decision-making skills. It is important that students do access support which is available to them throughout their pre-registration programme from personal tutors, clinical mentors, module leaders and also academic support so that they know what is expected of them and how to achieve.

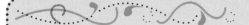

Chapter summary

The essence of this chapter has been to encourage you to consider what it means to be professional, recognise the key characteristics associated with being professional and understand how your behaviour, knowledge and actions impact on the perceived professional image of nursing. It is all too easy for us to forget the impact we as individuals can make to the standing and success of nursing.

It is also important to recognise that there is little doubt that the image of nursing has been subject to a wide range of influences and continues to evolve in light of ever-changing roles and responsibilities. Sadly, inaccurate and negative stereotypes continue to abound and representations of the role of the nurse remain distorted. The delivery of nursing care is a dynamic ever-changing process, requiring individual nurses and nursing as a profession to continue to advance if they are to live up to the demands and expectations of those who are receiving their care.

Activities: brief outline answers

Activity 2.2 (page 30)

Why is regulation necessary?

The primary purpose of regulation is to protect and promote the safety of the public by ensuring all registered nurses and midwives are properly qualified and competent to work in the UK. The NMC is the statutory regulatory body for nursing and midwifery.

Regulation is necessary to set standards of education, behaviour and ethics that nurses and midwives must meet. It also allows the regulatory body, that is, the NMC, to provide consistency and fairness when regulating practice and also when concerns about nurses who are unfit to practise as a result of ill health, poor performance and misconduct are raised. The NMC has the power to remove professionals from the register and prevent them from practising where they consider this to be in the best interests of public safety. In addition, the NMC, as part of the CHRE, is also responsible for shaping the ongoing development of regulatory processes for nursing and other healthcare professionals, thereby driving up standards.

Does regulation automatically confer professional status?

No. Regulation does not automatically confer professional status. Statutory regulation exists within both medicine, by the GMC, and nursing and midwifery, by the NMC. However, it is widely acknowledged that nursing retains a subordinate status within the medical hierarchy and, as discussed within the chapter, there is still dispute today as to whether nursing is a profession, since we do not have an exclusive body of knowledge.

Activity 2.4 (pages 34–5)

1. Two students using social networking sites

It is important to realise that how you behave on line can have an impact on whether you are able to qualify. As a student nurse it is important to be careful that what you get up to on the internet can compromise your fitness to practise. Anything posted online may end up in the public domain and could be read and/or viewed by members of the public. How you behave on line is not the same as doing what you like in private. Potentially in this situation if you are discussing learning experience you could be in breach of confidentiality and your integrity may also be brought into question. The protection of the public is paramount and such a situation would be investigated by the university's fitness to practise panel. Universities do provide guidance regarding social networking sites, so you do need to familiarise yourself with this.

The university is required at the end of training to sign a declaration of good health and character. Good character is based upon conduct, behaviour and attitudes that might bring the profession into disrepute. You can protect your online reputation by ensuring that you do set privacy and security settings; by treating all online conversations as if you were talking in public; by not posting information when you are under the influence of alcohol; and by not posting explicit information. It is also important to remember not to reveal personal information about yourself which could also put you at risk.

2. Student with 46 days uncertified absence due to sickness

The kind of things that you would need to consider in this situation is that the sickness would suggest that the student's health has deteriorated while they have been on the programme and/or that the sickness is a consequence of attempting to manage a different issue. Although in this situation it is the student's responsibility to advise either their personal tutor or programme leader of any changes in their health status, since they have not done so the educational institution would need to investigate the situation. If the sickness was due to a health problem, it may be necessary for the student to be referred to occupational health to see if they are fit to practise, and also to explore if any reasonable adjustments need to be made. If the absence is due to a different reason, it would be useful to explore that situation further and offer support as appropriate.

From a professional perspective, you need to consider whether the student has adhered to local rules and regulations re sickness and absence reporting and, if not, why not. You also need to consider whether the student's health is impacting upon their ability to practise safely and effectively. In this situation, the student has missed both theory and practice time, and would be required to demonstrate how they have made up this time. The NMC stipulates the number of hours of theory and practice a student must complete for each stage of their nursing preparation programme.

It is also important to bear in mind that educational institutions are required to make a declaration at the end of each student's training, stating that they are of good health and good character sufficient to ensure safe and effective practice. Good character is based on your conduct and, if the student has lied about illness, it would bring their honesty and integrity into question.

3. Student arrested for driving while over the legal alcohol limit

You will need to consider that if, during the pre-registration programme, a student receives a conviction or caution for any offence, this may impact on their good character and they must notify the university. If necessary, a fitness to practise panel will meet to make a decision about their suitability for practice.

Depending on the offence, the university may decide that it is willing to sign the declaration of good health and character at the end of training or it may decide that it is unable to sign; however, the student should be kept fully informed of any decisions made. In this situation, drinking and driving, it may also have implications for the student's future employment as a registered nurse if they wish to secure employment where the post holder is required to have a current driving licence.

Activity 2.9 (page 42)

Different standards of behaviour may be expected of you as a student nurse studying for both a professional and academic award from standards expected of other students who are studying solely for an academic award, because you are required to demonstrate fitness to practise as a nurse. You will be required to adhere to a code of professional conduct developed by your educational institute, which is based on the current NMC *Code* (2007a) and which provides you with benchmarks for behaviour.

When considering other healthcare professionals' codes of conduct, things that you may wish to take into account relate to the similarities and differences in:

* standards of conduct, performance and ethics;
* standards of proficiency;
* standards required for education and training;
* character and health;
* standards for continuing professional development.

Some of the common reasons why a student's fitness to practise may be questioned relate to behaviour within university, clinical practice settings and everyday life. These can include academic offences, such as plagiarism, a failure to meet the practice requirements of a learning experience, for example in terms of skills and communications, and professional behaviour, such as substance abuse, dishonesty and lack of integrity. Likewise, if there is a change in the student's health status or they receive a criminal conviction or caution, these may also preclude the student from fulfilling their professional responsibilities.

Further reading

Brown, J and Libberton, P (eds) (2007) *Principles of Professional Studies in Nursing*. Basingstoke: Palgrave Macmillan.

A useful text, which explores beliefs and values of nursing, management of care issues, evidence-based practice and clinical effectiveness.

Gobbi, M (2005) Nursing practice as a bricoleur activity: A concept explored. *Nursing Inquiry* 12(2): 117–25.

This article explores the debate surrounding the nature of nursing practice. It reflects on how learning and knowledge are developed by registered nurses, drawing on various bodies of evidence gained through education and practical experience in order to deal with the multitude of situations they encounter when dealing with the needs of individual patients.

Hart, C (2004) *Nurses and Politics: The impact of power and practice*. Basingstoke: Palgrave Macmillan.

A useful text, which offers insight into the links between politics and the development of nursing.

Useful websites

www.hpc-uk.org

Health Professions Council – regulator whose aim is to protect the public and currently regulates 13 healthcare professions.

www.icn.ch

International Council of Nurses website.

www.nhshistory.com

NHS history site run by Geoffrey Rivett.

www.nmc-uk.org

Website of the Nursing and Midwifery Council – the governing body for nurses and midwives.

www.rcn.org.uk

Website of the Royal College of Nursing – the professional association for nurses.

Chapter 3
Theories of nursing, and nursing as a caring activity

Carol Hall

NMC Standards for Pre-registration Nursing Education

This chapter will address the following competencies:

Domain 1: Professional values

2. All nurses must practise in a holistic, non-judgmental, caring and sensitive manner that avoids assumptions, supports social inclusion; recognises and respects individual choice; and acknowledges diversity. Where necessary, they must challenge inequality, discrimination and exclusion from access to care.

3. All nurses must support and promote the health, wellbeing, rights and dignity of people, groups, communities and populations. These include people whose lives are affected by ill health, disability, ageing, death and dying. Nurses must understand how these activities influence public health.

Domain 2: Communication and interpersonal skills

2. All nurses must use a range of communication skills and technologies to support person-centred care and enhance quality and safety. They must ensure people receive all the information they need in a language and manner that allows them to make informed choices and share decision making. They must recognise when language interpretation or other communication support is needed and know how to obtain it.

Domain 4: Leadership, management and team working

2. All nurses must systematically evaluate care and ensure that they and others use the findings to help improve people's experience and care outcomes and to shape future services.

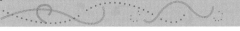

NMC Essential Skills Clusters

This chapter will address the following ESCs:

Cluster: Care, compassion and communication

1. As partners in the care process, people can trust a newly registered graduate nurse to provide collaborative care based on the highest standards, knowledge and competence.
6. People can trust the newly registered nurse to engage therapeutically and actively listen to their needs and concerns, responding using skills that are helpful, providing information that is clear, accurate, meaningful and free from jargon.

Cluster: Organisational aspects of care

11. People can trust the newly registered nurse to safeguard children and adults from vulnerable situations and support and protect them from harm.

Chapter aims

After reading this chapter, you will be able to:

- explore a personal philosophy of nursing as a caring activity from your own beliefs, values and understanding and from existing theoretical perspectives;
- understand key considerations relating to the fundamental nursing concepts of 'man', 'health', 'society' and 'nursing';
- describe how changes in the defining relationships between these concepts can offer different models of nursing practice;
- compare personal values with wider corporate philosophical positions relating to UK contemporary nursing;
- explain how an evidence base can be supported in delivering nursing in different nursing situations.

Introduction

The first two chapters have focused on the nature of nursing, and how it is defined as a profession by nurses and by others in society. In the next two chapters, the focus moves on, this time to explore the concept of nursing as an evidence-based, participative activity. This chapter will examine how the action of nursing is constructed, taking into consideration the ultimate goals of nursing, adopting the Henderson (1966) definition of optimum health for the individual or, if appropriate in the circumstances, a peaceful death. Consideration will also be given to the act of nursing within the environment in which it is carried out. Knowing what nursing is, and how it is defined as an activity, is essential when preparing to assess patients or clients and beginning to plan to deliver the nursing care they need.

Nursing as an activity may be defined differently in accordance with differing theoretical perspectives and foundation concepts. This is important for you to understand, as it enables some appreciation of why nursing in very different contexts with different activities may still nevertheless be considered to be nursing. As an example, a plan of care devised by a nurse working as part of a multidisciplinary surgical team within a large technology-led teaching hospital in the affluent Western world may be very different from that planned by one nurse working alone with a large number of patients in a small rural clinic in sub-Saharan Africa. The care planned for an individual with mental health needs living within a community or home setting is likely to be different again. Nursing care is influenced by many variables, including individual countries' legislation, professional influences, and resource requirements, and availability. It is also influenced by the vision for what is achievable in determining a healthy outcome, and by societal expectations.

This chapter will begin by encouraging you to explore your own beliefs about what a nurse must consider when preparing to assess, plan and deliver care for patients, and about what the role of the patient or client might be. You will be encouraged to consider the outcomes of nursing – what is health and what does health mean to you? This will be compared with other theoretical stances, enabling you to develop your understanding of the key components of nursing theory development through combining your personal experience and the knowledge gained from this chapter in developing a personal philosophy of nursing. You will also be encouraged to consider the impact of differences in societies on the kind of nursing care that may be needed and delivered.

The availability of resources and care environments will be explored, and also contemporary evidence, as it relates to the act of carrying out nursing. This consideration will be supported for you by glimpses of the past as well as by contemporary evidence – using classical 'models' of thinking identified by nursing theorists as they have tried to elicit the answers to these questions – as well as research findings when appropriate.

Throughout the chapter, you will be encouraged to draw your thinking together in creating your own plan for delivering care based on your current knowledge and reading, as well as your personal thinking and values. Towards the end of the chapter, it is important to think about how your philosophy can fit with the philosophies of institutions and of others involved in caring. Knowing your position in the context of others can enable you to deliver nursing practice knowledgeably with reflective insight, which can contribute to safe, effective and ethical practice. This will lead into Chapter 4, which will enable you to begin to assess, plan and deliver nursing care in a practical way.

Thinking about nursing – what are your values and beliefs and why are they important to you?

To explore your own 'philosophy' of nursing, you first need to begin to define your own ideas about nursing, and it is helpful to think about what the main components of nursing as an activity might be. It is also important to realise that, when developing your own philosophy, it is not only for your own benefit. Although this is important right now, in the future you are likely to have to convey your ideas to others. It is important, therefore, to think carefully about articulating your ideas. What will you say? How can you share your messages? We all think we know what we mean and communicate effectively in relation to nursing, but actually it is not as simple as that. Individual conceptions and definitions of the same terminology do differ and actually language is a very crude tool.

The next exercise uses the seemingly concrete concept of the word 'vehicle' in an activity to illustrate this problem. Don't worry that the exercise moves away from nursing briefly. It is just that defining 'vehicle' is clearer and easier to begin with than using the term 'nursing'. You will return to nursing afterwards.

Activity 3.1   *Reflection*

Take a piece of paper and draw upon it something that, for you, illustrates the word 'vehicle'.

If possible, get a friend or work colleague to do the same.

When you have finished this activity, spend a few minutes reflecting on your drawing and consider the following.

- Is this the only way you could have drawn a vehicle? If you have drawn a car, could you have done it differently? What does the word 'vehicle' actually mean? (As a human biologist you may have been justified in drawing some red blood cells, as the blood is a vehicle for the carriage of nutrients and waste materials.)
- Thinking about the different definitions of the term 'vehicle' – what are the commonalities? Think about the purpose and aim of the vehicle and what it basically must have in order to function.
- If we skip the biologist's theory for now and focus upon motor vehicles, it is possible to define the aim as movement of people or goods from one place to another. (The purpose, how many and where to and how fast may vary and this will affect your illustration.) It is also possible to identify some fundamental concepts that are essential in enabling effective function – means of propulsion, entry/exits, means of steering and stopping.

continued overleaf . . .

continued . . .

Now compare your vehicle with your colleague's version. Are they the same, or have you drawn a sports car and your colleague an aeroplane? One of the difficulties of using the term 'vehicle' is that it is a very broad concept and can mean different things to different people. The same basic premises are included in each vehicle but the relationship and functions of these will differ.

Finally consider – as your drawing currently exists – could you use it? What would it take to make it actually useful? We will come back to this question at the end of the chapter.

As this activity is based on your own observations, and as we will relate this example to nursing care delivery in the following text, there is no outline answer at the end of the chapter.

Applying and understanding nursing theory in delivering your care

In exactly the same way that you were asked to draw a picture of a vehicle in the above example, it is possible to consider the main components and relationships associated with the term 'nursing', and in doing so you will be following a long line of theorists going back at least as far as Florence Nightingale (1860) in her book, *Notes on Nursing: What it is and what is not*. Outside nursing, you are joining great philosophical thinkers, including Aristotle, Plato, Bacon, Kant and Descartes . . . Back to nursing, though, and after all this thinking, many theorists now have come to agree on the main components of 'nursing' as conceptualising practice by 'nurses' of caring for individuals in need of care (patients or clients) to achieve a particular goal of 'health' within a given environment and societal context. Just as your vehicle needed specific components in order to define it as a vehicle in the activity above, the components of 'nursing', 'man', 'health' and 'society' are well documented as key to defining nursing as a concept. These form the basis for discussion about what the action of nursing actually is, and although they are accepted by many and are pragmatically useful in the context of this chapter, it is important to know that even these have been challenged (McKenna, 1997; McKenna and Slevin, 2008). This underlines the complexity of defining nursing as an activity.

If you do accept these, however, just as in the vehicle example the questions continue – the definitions of the role of the nurse, the role of the patient, the context of what health is, and the impact and role of society and the environment are all debated in the nursing literature. Such debates and their outcomes form historical and practical differences in the ways that nursing is delivered. They also form a difference in the perceived and expected outcome of nursing, defined in this work as a concept of 'health'. Although the concepts are agreed, the ways in which each is defined using individual values and beliefs differ, and the relationships between the concepts also differ.

At first, it may help to think about a typical scenario of nursing as identified in your experience and using this, thinking about why you have chosen to become a nurse. What are the activities of nursing? Who is involved and where does it take place in your scenario? This may take you back to your activities in Chapter 1, which relate to what you believe about being a nurse, but it should make you think more widely about the beliefs and values you have. The following case studies might help with your ideas.

Case studies

'I am 19 years old and a first-year student nurse in a university school of nursing in London, UK. I have just attended my first learning experience in a children's surgical ward, where children attend needing a range of different operative procedures. I have not worked in nursing before, but I have done some voluntary work abroad in an American summer camp for children. From my experience, I believe that nursing is about caring for patients and their families throughout their time in hospital, even though their stay might be very short. I need to make sure that the children are able to have their operations safely and successfully through making sure they have everything they need and they understand the care. I know it is important to ensure that pre- and post-operative procedures are carried out and the right equipment is available. From my knowledge of nursing, I know that surgical nursing in hospital is only one aspect of caring performed by nurses and there are many more. My values are about putting the patient and their family first and about being a professional person in the care I give. For me, health is when patients and their families can go home and no longer need hospital services.'

'I am 38 years old and a new student nurse with no practice learning experience yet undertaken in my course. I have come into a pre-registration nursing education course from being a care worker in a care of the elderly home for many years. I had to study an access course to refresh my study as I left school a long time ago. I have a family myself; my two children are teenagers now and I care for my mother, who is elderly and who lives near us. From my experience, I believe nursing is about caring for patients at every stage of life to give them independence in a safe manner and to allow them to participate in social activities. Many of the people I have cared for have had physical disabilities as a result of their age, or have dementia. My values are about increasing my knowledge of the best ways to care for people to offer them dignity, independence and the best quality of life. For me, health is about being able to participate fully in every aspect of your life.'

Create your own personal pen portrait case study like the ones above. When you are doing this, you are beginning to espouse your beliefs and values and effectively you are beginning to draw some ideas together that will develop through this chapter into your personal 'philosophy' of nursing. Look at the 'Concept summary' box below to understand a little more about nursing philosophy and theory construction.

Concept summary: Philosophy

What does 'philosophy' actually mean? How does philosophy fit with 'ontology' and 'epistemology', and what has this got to do with nursing and where does nursing theory fit?

Philosophy is defined by Fawcett (1992, cited in McKenna and Slevin, 2008) and supported by McKenna as being '*a statement of beliefs and values about the world, a perspective on human beings and their world and an approach to the development of knowledge*' (1997, p6; McKenna and Slevin, 2008).

Sub-branches of philosophical thinking include:

- epistemology – related to a concept of knowing: what the knowledge is surrounding nursing and what can be known about nursing;
- logical reasoning and thinking;
- ethics – concerned with standards of conduct;
- aesthetics – concerned with actualising the best personal reality;
- politics – concerned with the values and beliefs associated with regulation of society;
- metaphysics – concerned with the nature of our existence on the grandest scale.
  (Adapted from Chitty and Black, 2007)

Ontology follows from the concept of metaphysics and defines a concept of 'being': *In relation what could (or should) nursing be?* (Brown and Gobbi, 2007, p10). Nursing theory – in its simplest definition, a theory brings together all of the above and a *model* assists by offering a means for the theory to be illustrated and discussed with others (like a blueprint for reality). Theories can be designed and then imposed on a situation and tested to see if they work (deductive theories) or they can be generated from observing practice and writing down the observations about what works (inductive theories). They can be brought together on the basis of a philosophy and derive from it, or they could be brought together pragmatically from many different theoretical stances (eclectic theories). Finally, the extent to which a theory has been tested and empirically validated will determine what *type* of theory it is.

It is perhaps a little strange to be thinking about philosophy and its related concerns when trying to examine what a nurse actually does. However, all nursing decisions that are carried out include values determined in the heads of the people who are undertaking the activity of nursing at the time. This is the case from the highest strategic level, when considering documents such as *Modernising Nursing Careers* (DH, 2006), to the newest student trying to develop rationalised directions and reasons for giving care. These are combined with the best available evidence, using research, evaluative studies, best practice examples and policy work, to support future directions in nursing. It is important for you to do the same and begin to generate an understanding of your own personal philosophy of nursing. By writing this down, you will be taking a snapshot picture of your perspective now, given what you know and believe today. Knowing what you think about nursing will help you in delivering and discussing care that you may plan for patients, and see where your values and beliefs may differ from other people's ideas or from the ideas of an institution or an employer. A personal philosophy of nursing is also a useful tool to keep in your portfolio, because it will enable you to look back and reflect in future, to see whether your values have remained the same over time or whether they have changed as you progress through your career.

Activity 3.2	*Critical thinking*

Under the headings of 'man (patient)', 'society', 'health' and 'nursing', try to draft out your current beliefs and values. Use your pen portrait to add ideas.

- Try to think about the roles of the patient and the nurse, and what nursing should be, and what the best nursing might be (using the ideas of aesthetics and ontology).
- Use your knowledge of nursing, found in evidence-based documents you have read so far, to support your own ideas and generate personal knowledge for your practice (using epistemological stances).
- Think about the moral and ethical positions of nursing as an activity – can you see any challenges in this?
- Does politics play a part in defining nursing?

Take time also to reflect on your ability to undertake this activity. What processes of learning are you using and what are your thinking methods? Have you read around and adopted one person's theory or are you doing this from the heart, collecting many different ideas from a range of sources? How do you know what you know? What have you learnt through the activity? These thoughts are important now. You will be considering a few of the thoughts of eminent theorists in relation to their ideas about nursing. Keep your philosophy close by and reflect on it as you read the next section.

As this activity is based on your own thoughts, there is no outline answer at the end of the chapter. However, the following discussion in the text will offer many answers.

How 'man', 'health', 'society' and 'nursing' are used to think about nursing

The components of 'man', 'health', 'society' and 'nursing' underpin mission statements, patients' rights documents and guidelines for good practice in healthcare more broadly. The next section is going to explore different ways in which the concepts of man, health, society and nursing have been defined and applied by others. This is important because changing the emphasis and nature of these concepts can change the way the nursing care is delivered. This helps to explain also how different care delivery systems function. A clear example of this can be seen when comparing the NHS system in the UK with the US system, which relies on patient insurance. Such a radical difference in the funding environment for healthcare affects the rights of the patients to receive care and the roles of nurses in delivering nursing. These components also help you to consider how and why you deliver nursing in particular way.

To consider some different examples of nursing care delivery in more detail, some ideas based on those of a few very classical nursing theorists will be used for illustration. These early theorists were stark in their thinking and their work can enable clarity through drawing on the most basic premises of their arguments. It is fair to say that the theories presented are simplified from the original to offer illustration only and the original theories should be explored for greater detail. Further, many more nurses have developed theories since these earlier ones, offering new ideas and 'models' for the delivery of nursing care, and you will find them in your reading.

Nursing is also not a pure science, as the profession does accept theoretical positions and models from outside the discipline of nursing where it is useful to do so. Two specific models from outside nursing can be found in this chapter – Becker's Health Belief Model (Becker and Maiman, 1975), which emanates from public health medicine but uses behavioural theory, and the European Resuscitation Council algorithm for basic life support and resuscitation (ERC, 2010), which has a background within medicine – but in your practice you will find many more. From a historical perspective, there is also a traditional perspective of the 'medical model', which was used by nurses in the UK until the mid-1970s and remains influential today. There is not the space to address the full complexity of any individual theory in this chapter, but these can be found in a summary by Brown and Libberton (2007).

It is important to remember always that the nursing theorists being discussed in the next section are basically nurses trying to make sense of their situation in order to justify and improve the care they wanted to give to their patients. (This is what you have to do as well, and are doing in developing your own philosophy.) Look at the weblinks to find out more about these nursing theorists as people and their ideas.

Pen portrait: Callista Roy

Dr Callista Roy is a professor and theorist currently working at the William F Connell School of Nursing, Boston. In her early career as a children's nurse and as a committed Christian, Roy realised her model from consideration of the scientific elements of adaptation she observed in the world of nursing.

Roy noted that the relationships between a person, their thoughts, feelings and expectations, as well as their environment, mitigated adaptive or coping responses. She reasoned that such interaction between systems could promote or weaken an individual's capacity for coping and adaptation. In illness, therefore, the individual's capacity to adapt or cope with the situation could be facilitated by effecting a kind of nursing that took acount of, and helped to create, an optimum environment, both physically and mentally, for the individual.

(www.bc.edu/schools/son/faculty/theorist/Roy_Adaptation_Model.html)

Pen portrait: Dorothea Orem

Dr Dorothea Orem was born in 1914 in Maryland. She qualified as a nurse in the 1930s in America, and began publishing in relation to her theoretical view of nursing in the 1950s, continuing to contribute to nursing theory development until she died in 2007 at the age of

93. In her self-care theory (1999), Dr Orem identified that the relationship between nurses and their patients and clients was pivotal in the way that they could be helped to achieve health. Orem began by suggesting that patients were essentially self-caring and able individuals who, in the event of ill health, suffered identifiable deficits. The nurse role would be to understand and support these deficits and at the same time enable the patient to continue to be self-caring in every other way. In time, and with appropriate treatment, the patient would be able to return to independence, or the capacity that needed care could be transferred to an appropriate agency. This approach was initially heavily criticised for being linguistically complex and difficult to use with those who relied on others for their care (such as children), but it developed dynamically over the years and is now established with a scholarly following and supportive research. The principle philosophy held by Orem of the view of the patient as independent is an important perspective, as illustrated in this chapter.

(**www.scdnt.com**)

Pen portrait: Hildegard Peplau

Hildegard Peplau was born in 1909 and became a nurse in psychiatry during the 1940s following a broader career in general nursing. She was one of the first of the contemporary theorists in nursing, drawing her expertise from working with psychologists, including Erich Fromm. She used her theory to advocate changes in mental health practice, from the custodial care existent at the time to the provision of a therapeutic and relational environment. Peplau focused on the part played by emotional health and the contribution of nursing as a role, which meant negotiating with patients to determine their needs and to establish treatment and care. This model was widely accepted in mental health areas, as the benefits of seeing nursing differently from a purely physical concept of caring were clearly evident.

(**publish.uwo.ca/~cforchuk/peplau/hpcb.html**)

Pen portrait: Nancy Roper

Nancy Roper was a UK theorist born in Cumberland in 1918. She qualified in children's nursing and general nursing and then nurse education, before researching and writing about a theory for practice as part of her Master's in Philosophy studies in the 1970s (Marriner et al., 2006). Roper is most famous for the model of nursing she subsequently derived with two other UK theorists, Winifred Logan and Alison Tierney. Their philosophy was simply based on the notion of the patient performing a range of essential 'activities of living'. The nurse could assess these and determine the patient's needs based upon their independence or need for care in relation to each activity. This model has underpinnned most modern pathways of nursing in the UK and elements of this are commonly found within assessment and care planning documentation in the UK today. It is commended for its simplicity and ease of use, which has contributed to its prevalence in UK healthcare settings.

(www.independent.co.uk/news/obituaries/nancyroper543782.html)

Defining the role of the nurse in the patient or client relationship

The last two chapters have extensively considered how nursing is influenced professionally and legally, and by the media stereotypes portrayed. However, this has not described what nurses actually do in respect of giving care to patients. It is true that nurses must work ethically, professionally and legally, and in a skilled way to make sure that patients receive the most appropriate care, but this says nothing at all about their perceived role in practice. Three theorists identified quite different roles for the nurse in their early works and these are worth exploring. It is fair to say that later works enabled a blending of these positions, and now each position may be used by you at different times in the delivery of your nursing care.

The nurse as a 'doer' or 'intervener' – caregiver and patient as a passive recipient of care

This position was defined originally by Henderson (1966) from original medical models of care and was adopted subsequently by Roper et al. (1980) in their Activities of Living Model adapted from Henderson's original ideology for the UK nursing market. The focus of the patient as a passive recipient was heavily criticised, but fitted well with the period in which it was originally developed (1966), when care was dominantly in hospital settings with a strong medical influence. The model also reflected the media image of the nurse, who was portrayed as being subservient to medical staff but in control of patients. In later works, this limitation of the role of the nurse was recognised and the notion of the patient as being placed along a continuum of dependence to independence was considered more in relation to the nurse's corresponding role. However, the stark original position of Henderson's nursing role remains important, because the way in which patients are cared for will still influence the way in which they behave, even today. For many patients, being in need of health services is frightening and worrying, and a care setting can be alien and strange. The instinctively safe passive patient role, which seems to allow the experts to do their work, is a tempting and reasonable response. For the professional, the mystique of the professional decision, historically much associated with medicine, may be viewed as a source of expertise by the public and something commanding respect.

One of the difficulties associated with the nurse as a 'doer' approach when this is taken to the extreme, however, is that patients may return to their homes less healthy than when they attended the care setting in the first place! In terms of best practice, also, the patient's role in understanding, participating in and challenging the care they receive is important, and this is difficult if they are passive recipients of care, as in the following case study, for example.

Case study

Mr Peter Brown was 82 years old and lived independently in his own home. His wife had died some years before and he had managed to care for himself independently since this time. One day on a shopping trip to the local town, Mr Brown tripped over the edge of the kerb and fell, injuring his ankle and hitting his head. He was taken to the local hospital, where it was decided that it would be appropriate for him to be admitted for observation. Although his injuries were slight, during his stay in hospital Mr Brown was quiet and demonstrated some mild signs of disorientation, so his stay was extended. The nurses provided care for him. They washed him and dressed him, and provided meals for him. They supplied him with a wheelchair and wheeled him to the dining room, because it took him a long time to walk. Each time they offered care to Mr Brown they told him that they 'were just going to wash/dress/etc. him' and asked his permission. Mr Brown thought the nurses were very caring, but he really wanted to go home to his community. He thought that the nurses knew best and waited for them to provide his care without question.

Mr Brown recovered slowly and physically became well enough to return home. However, he lost his skills of independence while in hospital and his occupational therapy assessments suggested that he would be unable to live on his own safely again, even with support from community nurses. Finally, Mr Brown was assessed for a place in a care home 20 miles from where he used to live.

While the nurses cared for Mr Brown's every need, the role of the nurse as the doer in this situation may have been detrimental to him. By doing everything, the nurses took away Mr Brown's independence and he lost his capacity to manage for himself. Even though the nurses asked Mr Brown's permission, the language that they used implied that they were 'doers'. Using phrases like 'we are just going to wash/dress/etc. you' implied the dominant role of the nurse and correspondingly the passivity of the patient, even when permission was asked.

Now consider some alternatives. As shown above, Orem (1985) designed a theory that identified the concept of the 'self-caring' patient. In this model, the role of the nurse related to one of supporter and facilitator, providing care as an agency for the more usual self-care, which assisted the patient only when it was clear in the assessment that the patient could not care for themselves. In the case of Peter Brown, nurses using Orem's approach would only offer to assist with elements that he could not do and the expectation would be that, in all other aspects, he would be self-caring. Mr Brown would wash and dress himself and would walk to the dining room slowly. The nurses' role in supporting Mr Brown would be by ensuring he was able to self-care effectively in the circumstances and encourage the self-caring role through reassurance, support and education. While it is sometimes difficult to see how Orem's model can work effectively – in situations where critical care is needed and the patient is totally dependent – for Mr Brown this approach could have been useful. Care would have assessed with a focus on what he was able to do and the nurses would support him only in the areas he needed rather than doing everything.

A further alternative, identified by Hildegard Peplau, took the concept of patient empowerment even further. Peplau (1952) suggested that the patient should be responsible for deciding what care they needed and negotiating the care needed with the nurse who responded, ultimately empowering the patient to self-determination. This theory turns the concept of the nurse as a doer on its head and creates a situation where potentially the nurse may play a fairly passive role, although the concept of the nurse as an advocate is strongly featured in this work. Such a philosophy of care is particularly appropriate in relation to the nurse–patient relationship in mental health settings, where empowerment for independence and increasing self-esteem is very important.

Activity 3.3   *Research and evidence-based practice*

Take the time to visit a healthcare setting or care learning experience where nursing care is taking place. Observe the delivery of nursing and evaluate the following.

* What are the nurses actually doing?
* How do they respond to their clients? What language and non-verbal communication is used and what does it imply to you?
* Are the nurses acting as doers or facilitators, or do they change their position in different circumstances?
* Who decides about the care that needs to be given?
* Ask yourself: Is the approach used a good one for those needing care? Could a different approach be used? What effect would changing the role of the nurse or client have had in this situation?

As this activity is based on your own observations, there is no outline answer at the end of the chapter.

The nurse as an advocate in care and patients' rights to consent to care given

While the theorists have considered the role of the nurse in a very practical way and reflected this in the corresponding role of the patient or client, the role of the nurse as an advocate has been addressed separately in the nursing literature. Indeed, it has even been debated whether nurses can ever effectively advocate for patients and, in the event, whether they should actually do so. This is because the very role of advocacy requires nurses to exert professional opinion and influence in the interests of the patient. However, taken to a logical conclusion, the concept of what is good for the patient is decided by the nurse advocate in their professional opinion – if patients are to be able to have the freedom to take decisions about their health and, as such, be empowered, there must be a careful balance struck between the nurse's role as advocate, and her or his role in enabling patients to give their consent in an informed way. Clearly, however, there are times when patient advocacy by the nurse is necessary, occurring when the patient is unable for health or age reasons to take their own decisions, or where there is no close living relative, or where life is at risk and informed consent is not possible.

Concept summary: Advocacy and the nurse as advocate

Advocacy is:

- a process whereby a nurse or other healthcare professional provides a patient with the information to make certain decisions, usually related to some aspect of the patient's healthcare;
- a method by which patients, their families, attorneys, health professionals and citizen groups can work together to develop programmes that ensure the availability of high-quality healthcare for a community;
- pleading a cause on behalf of another, such as a nurse pleading for better care of a patient or for the patient's desires to be honoured.

(Adapted from Mosby, 2009)

The concept of patient empowerment is a critical concern in our society today and Peplau's theory holds relevance much more widely in contemporary nursing than just in mental health settings. Indeed, the concept of patient choice is perceived by healthcare policymakers to be essential within the UK health system. A example of this relates to the Darzi Inquiry (DH, 2008b), which spent time considering what patients really wanted from a modern NHS. Lord Darzi sought the opinions of the public on a grand scale, enabling them to have a say about the kind of care they wished to receive, and challenged the NHS to deliver from the grass-roots of local care delivery to the highest echelons of Government. Lord Darzi's main aim was to empower patients by helping to make healthcare provision recognisable and closer to public ideology.

Nursing and a concept of health

Health has been defined in a range of ways over a long time. It is important for nursing and indeed for other allied healthcare professions that an understanding of the meaning of health is attained, because it is the goal or outcome to which nursing should aspire. If patients achieve health, their need for nursing changes. However, determining a definition of health is not as simple as it seems. This is because health is a concept that is frequently determined by the person for whom it is an issue, and one person's health can easily be someone else's ill health!

Scenarios

- *You fall in an accident, and injure your ankle. It is not painful, but it does give way sometimes when you walk on it and you have resorted to using a walking stick for support. Would you say that you are healthy or that your health is not complete? Look at the WHO definition below to help with your decision.*
- *Now think about Sarah. She is the same age as you, but had her foot amputated as a child following an episode of meningococcal meningitis, which left her with tissue necrosis. She walks with assistance. When Sarah is asked whether she is healthy she replies that she is.*

Reflect on these two scenarios – at first consideration, it could be suggested that Sarah is not optimally healthy, as she has an illness-induced injury. Using the WHO definition, however, by Sarah's own perception she has complete physical, mental and social well-being, albeit without the existence of her foot. For you, however, your perception of your situation may be quite different, as the symptoms you have could indicate for you infirmity and an assault on your usual physical well-being.

Concept summary: Defining health

Probably the best known global definition of health is that of the World Health Organization (WHO). WHO defined health as being a state of complete physical, mental and social well-being and not merely the absence of disease or infirmity (1948, p100). Although this is an old definition, it remains commonly cited and is accepted by many as a truly global definition of health. WHO has never updated this statement and it remains on its website (**www.who.int**).

Within the WHO definition, it is also possible to see that a peaceful death is an acceptable goal within nursing in cases where health is not a feasible option. This is because WHO presents a definition in which the relationship between well-being and disease is challenged. While health could be the absence of infirmity and disease, this is insufficient without the complete state of physical, mental and social well-being. Conversely, it is argued that, even if you have disease or infirmity, it may be possible to have a sense of physical, mental and social well-being if you are pain free and able to live as you want to. This concept was adopted by Henderson (1966) in her theory and subsequently remains within the more recent Roper et al. (2000) model based on activities of living, and it is critical when considering the work of nursing, especially in relation to terminal care for patients and their families, either immediately resulting from acute events such as fatal accidents or illnesses, or in relation to longer-term palliative care situations where intervention for recovery to a state of health is identified as being unrealistic. Such planning can also be extended to other disciplines and pathways for effective care can be created. An example is included within the *Integrated Multi-agency Care Pathways for Children with Life-threatening and Life-limiting Conditions*, which allow consideration of multidisciplinary care for children in such circumstances (ACT, 2004).

The relationship between patients and their health

Empowerment in health

The concept of empowerment is critically important when exploring the relationship between patients or clients and their health. How patients are perceived or defined by others and, importantly, by themselves will define their response to illness and to the treatment that they receive. This feature also should be considered when planning any kind of health promotion activity, because for clients to be proactive in managing their health requires a realisation that the relationship between clients and their health is multifaceted, but requires appropriate support by the healthcare recipients as well as the providers.

To understand the concept of health more, it is also important to consider the ways in which patients become 'patients' and what defines them. If you look at evidence from the early social sciences, it is clear that patients are able to take on a 'sick' role. Talcott Parsons' (1951) concept of sickness as a role is documented extensively in the classical behavioural literature and complements work done that relates to health belief and health planning (Becker and Maiman, 1975; Tones and Tilford, 2001; Tones and Green, 2004). This role is identified with how patients see themselves and how they are treated by others, and this applies more widely than simply to the patient in the hospital bed. Use this link to a free, reusable learning object to find out more: **www.ucel.ac.uk/shield/parsons/Default.html**

Activity 3.4 — *Reflection*

Think back to a time when you were not feeling well at school or work and wanted to go home.

- How did you convey this to others?
- What differences were there in the way you behaved?
- How did others behave towards you?

A friend phones you the next day – you have taken the day off as you are still not able to work much but you are feeling better. What do you say – do you still play the sick role or do you identify that you are feeling better now?

- You might have said that you spoke to them or behaved differently from usual, or that others advised you to go home on hearing your situation – thus giving you 'permission' to play the 'sick' role.
- Where clients in your care are concerned, they may already feel that they have permission to play the sick role, and have their own perceptions about what that means, but they may receive some cues from you and may also need permission to participate in their own care depending on their expectations.

continued overleaf ...

---

continued . . . •••

- Think also about the cues that may indicate a 'sick' role – we frequently encourage hospital patients to dress in their nightwear during the day, but ask yourself – is this always needed? What messages are being sent to the patient and to those in contact with them? How do you feel when in your nightwear during daytime? Think also about the role of hair care and hygiene in promoting self-esteem and a sense of well-being.

As this activity is based on your own observation, there is no outline answer at the end of the chapter.

If Orem's (1985) Self-care Deficit Theory is used to illustrate an alternative position in relation to the Peter Brown scenario (see page 61), the nurse would assess him in terms of what he could do for himself, what assistance he might need and in what areas. Using this belief about nursing, the focus espoused encourages the patient to self-care as far as possible and receive support from nurses only in order to help themselves. While Orem has been criticised for her jargonistic writing, described by some as 'Oremese' because it is so difficult to understand, her philosophical stance around self-caring patients is well respected.

Activity 3.5   *Critical thinking*

On the NHS 'Go Smoke Free' website, look up the link for the video clip about Gary Lucy (**http://smokefree.nhs.uk/real-life-quitters/gary-lucy/index.php**).

The video clip shows a nurse helping a patient (Gary) to plan a path of care that will help him to stop smoking. Think about the relationship between the patient and his health, and the relationship between the patient and the nurse in this situation.

It is clear that the patient is empowered in this relationship with his nurse. The nurse gives him control, through asking him about what his ideas are for stopping smoking. Gary is advised about the measures that are there to support him and to enable him to measure his progress towards his goal of 'health' – which in this case means stopping smoking. For Gary, health is something that is a very personal goal, and, in order to get the support he needs, he has had to make the first move, that of attending for help. He explains his motivations for stopping and these are used by the nurse to continue to empower Gary, thus offering a model of health that is firmly focused upon the patient.

As this activity is based on your own reflection and observations, there is no outline answer at the end of the chapter.

In Activity 3.5, health is very much something that can be seen as an active outcome related to an empowering relationship. The patient, Gary, is actively encouraged to assess his own needs and to consider a plan of action that will meet these effectively.

The nurse's role is one of support and facilitation, and of realisation of resources to ensure that the goal of health is met. When considering health in this context, the assumption is that the resources to meet this health need are available and that the patient will be able to receive them freely if he decides with the nurse that this is what is needed. The environment is conducive to promoting optimum health, because it is feasible. While this approach mirrors a philosophy espoused by Hildegard Peplau (1952), as discussed earlier, in this scenario the outcome goal of health must be achievable or renegotiable, and the patient must be empowered to access the care and subscribe to a number of conditions. The healthcare environment must be one where realistic resources to achieve the goal of health are available and accessible.

Nursing the patient and health empowerment

It is important to recognise that the social context for health is dynamic and constantly changing and not every patient can look forward to the opportunities identified within the video clip relating to Gary. It is true that many patients today have more opportunities than ever before to be empowered by information and to know their rights and complain if they feel that their rights have not been sufficiently met. The use of the web and email, as well as touch screens and TVs within surgeries and public places, has made a difference to opportunities to gain information about health needs and the appropriate care that may be needed or given. Consequently, some patients are much more aware of their needs and can ask for treatments or refuse them, and some can use the media to make their views known and express their concerns about injustice. But you cannot assume this knowledge is there for everyone and in nursing there is also a major role not only of advocacy, as we have already described, but of enabling patients to access the care environment optimally. Older people, poorer people and people from different cultures are particularly vulnerable, as they are often not able to access the same media as others and sometimes have different perceptions of their role in healthcare as being more dependent upon the authority of nursing or medical staff. Nurses must have an appreciation of culturally and spiritually sensitive care when working with their patients, as well as assessing abilities and capacities for access to healthcare. It makes no difference if the best healthcare facilities lie in a brand new health centre, if the population who need the facilities either cannot or will not access them. This consideration relates back to those identified in Becker's Health Belief Model.

As a critique, it is difficult to achieve patient empowerment if given assumptions about the patient or about resources within the environment for care cannot be made. We have already noted this in relation to the discussions about the role of patients in their health and the nurse's role within this, but let us now explore the relationship between health and the environment or society where nursing might take place.

Health and the care environment

First, consider the above scenario about Gary Lucy. Compare this scenario to the perceptions of Florence Nightingale in her works on hospitals in the 1850s and 1860s. Nightingale offered a very early consideration of the patient in relation to his or her environment when she wrote *Notes on Nursing: What it is and what it is not* in 1859. Nightingale identified that it is not always possible to have a pill for every ill, and subsequently the truth of this has been demonstrated in many ways, which causes ethical as well as practical dilemmas within nursing, even today. To illustrate this further in relation to today's world, consider the concept of 'hygiene'. In 1869, Nightingale identified the benefits of good hygiene and good ventilation in reducing the spread of infection in hospitals. At this time there were no antibiotics and infection was a common problem, because standards of hygiene among patients and nurses alike were often poor, driven by poor environments for care with limited facilities, resources and knowledge. Nightingale's response in adapting the work of nurses in maintaining patient hygiene, ventilation and nutrition was critical in adapting environments towards the goal of optimum health.

If we fast-forward to the new millennium in the UK, past an age when antibiotics were discovered and used extensively to treat patients with a range of disorders, we enter the contemporary healthcare environment. Today, infections such as *MRSA* and *C. diff.* have become problematic in acute hospital settings and community homes alike, and intervening with medicines is challenging because of drug resistance. Once again nurses are challenged to consider their role in providing a better environment for patient care through careful handwashing and cleansing of clinical areas in order to protect patients from hospital-acquired infections (HAIs). With the publication of the *Essence of Care* benchmarks (DH, 2001) and the NMC pre-registration requirements for assessment in clinical skills relating to aseptic technique and medicines administration, providing an optimum environment for care is priority and beliefs about the importance of the nurse's role in ensuring an optimum environment for health are also evident in national policy. To open this consideration more widely and consider a global picture, WHO identified in their 2008 annual report, *Primary Health Care: 'Now more than ever'* that, although global health is improving, there are many countries in sub-Saharan Africa where babies and children continue to die because of malnutrition and poor hygiene, accidents and poor health provision. These are all preventable, given education and minimal resources.

Given the above situations, it is useful to think more widely about how the adaptation of care environments can contribute to promoting optimum health, both globally and in the UK, and Nightingale's original considerations still have utility even though the contexts of care are different.

Nurses are fundamental in manipulating the environment for care and Nightingale was not the only theorist who identifed the benefits of this kind of consideration. Think about the care of critically ill or injured patients and consider the following case study.

Case study

Joseph is 23 and a keen surfer. He spends as much time as he can on the beach at all times of year. On this occasion, Joseph is surfing in the autumn when there are no lifeguards around. He leaves the sea and collapses at the top of the beach not far from where you are out walking your dog. He has not drowned, but his breathing has stopped and on closer assessment he has no pulse. You have to do something and you use your skills learnt in basic life support as a new nurse to try to help him.

Following the ABC resuscitation guidance you learnt in school (e.g. European Resuscitation Council (ERC), 2010), you manage to begin to resuscitate Joseph, at the same time calling for help to others on the beach. Your efforts are successful. An ambulance takes Joseph to hospital and all is well. (**www.resus.org.uk/pages/faqALS.htm**)

continued opposite . . .

continued . . .

Think about your actions in this scenario. What were you actually doing? Upon reflection, can you identify the philosophical basis of the care you were giving to Joseph?

There is a brief outline answer at the end of the chapter.

Use of the resuscitation framework (ERC, 2010) offers similarity to the deliberations of the aforementioned theorist, Callista Roy. In Roy's (1976) theory, the patient was seen as having both internal and external homeostatic environmental systems, whereby balance is critical in enabling health in a wide range of situations. While this may sound strange, thinking about maintaining balance between internal and external systems can be helpful. For example, Roy's deliberations about the maintenance of homeostasis, or homeostatic balance within internal systems, work well in the above scenario. Your role as a nurse in this view is in manipulating the patient's internal environment to achieve the required outcome of health. However, you could also think about your actions in a different way. You could identify yourself as a nurse and the 'doer', and the patient as being on a continuum of dependence to independence (at this moment, dependent), and the action as being one that enables patient independence in the usual activities of breathing and maintaining a safe environment. This espouses the briefest consideration of the definition of the nurse within the model described by Roper et al. (1980). While many other theories have assessment mechanisms that would work in this situation and offer considerations that are useful, ultimately, in this situation the care you gave would need to be the same as it is in an emergency and you need to do whatever is best to save a life. Away from this event, however, it is useful to consider, understand and evaluate alternatives to be applied appropriately in given situations. Reflection on other ways of thinking offers insight and opportunities for evaluative practice.

In this chapter, you have explored some different situations that potentially reflect a need for different solutions. These included differences in the definition of the relative importance of the patient, the nurse, the care environment and the ultimate perception of health as a goal. To illustrate the possible alternative care mechanisms, some views from different nursing philosphies have been described. While you can use theorists' work to explore these differences, the final decision about your personal philosophy in delivering nursing care is your choice, and will impact upon the areas where you seek employment and the types of work you choose to do. All of these ideas must work together as a series of tools for you to draw upon in your thinking about your nursing.

Critical discussion: do models and theories in nursing work?

We will now look at the importance of dynamism in theory development and philosophical inquiry – and how lack of it may lead to abandonment.

Up to now you have considered the value of philosophies in nursing and explored your own beliefs. You have considered the fundamental elements of nursing and some of the relationships as they exist between these, and you have explored an example of the contemporary UK position, reflecting on the beliefs held in creating documents offering guidance defining nursing and in relation to the rights of patients in the UK. Finally, it is important to consider the different types of theory and the practical uses of these within nursing. It is important to critique the relative benefits and the limitations in order to consider how you might use the information gained in this chapter to best effect in your practice.

A brief critique of the use of theory and the different types found

Some nursing theories are considered to be conceptual (a description of the main concepts used in practice, but not tested using research to see if the theory works in delivering care). Others have empirical elements – they have been researched and developed in light of the evidence. Nurse theorists also work in one of two main ways in developing their theories – they can write about their own observations from within practice and develop these over time, which is known as inductive thinking (Cormack and Reynolds, 1992). This is a bit like the development of most new cars today, which are often generated from existing models and improved rather than starting afresh. Alternatively, a completely new theory might be developed and applied to practice to see if it would work, which is known as deductive thinking (Cormack and Reynolds, 1992). (Going back to cars, these are the 'concept' models.) An example of an inductive model can be seen in the Nottingham Model (Smith, 1995) for children's nursing, while Nightingale's model of nursing focused on building and adapting care environments to improve care outcomes, which was a new and radical way to consider nursing care delivery at the time.

While both of these kinds of theories use existing evidence to underpin the decisions taken and to justify their use, the discussion relating to the philosophical position and theory type is far less clear. Indeed, there is discussion about whether highly conceptual overarching style theories (sometimes identified as grand or global theories) and their subsequent models can actually improve delivery of nursing in practice or whether they more simply serve to inform practitioners about different ways of thinking (McKenna, 1997; McKenna and Slevin, 2008; Pesut and Johnson, 2008). Further, the number of theories that have included rigorous empirical testing of their efficacy in improving clinical practice is fairly limited.

Conclusion

In conclusion, it is critical to realise that continuing consideration of philosophies, theories and models is essential as nursing, as a knowledge-based profession, develops to meet new needs, for they do enable alternative thinking and consideration to be included within the practical work of nurses.

Indeed, more work is needed to evaluate the effectiveness of commonly applied theories and to modify ideas. Such critical evaluation and thinking can allow nurses to wonder about future possibilities and redesign practice to meet future needs (Pesut and Johnson, 2008). An example of critical evaluation in this area is illustrated well by Timmins and Horan (2007), in their work on the use of Orem's (2001) Self-care Deficit Theory in coronary care units. Timmins and Horan use the appraisal to consider the utility of the theory in practice, but even they recognise contemporary limitations relating to the lack of use and evaluation in practice. In light of this critique, it would appear that nursing is entering an interesting period in relation to nursing theory, where evaluation of practice in relation to theory is likely to be important in order to progress nursing ideology in a systematic way.

For you, gaining a broad understanding of the relationships defined within theoretical models is important – not because you will necessarily use one or another model of care exclusively (or if you do, you may do this because your employer may direct you anyway because, as we have already seen with the vehicle scenario, it is important to have a team thinking along similar lines), but because it is important to think about how you approach your care delivery on an individual basis and for you to be able to consider and articulate alternatives.

Activity 3.6   *Research and reflection*

Have a look at:

- *Defining Nursing* (RCN, 2003) on **www.rcn.org.uk/__data/assets/pdf_file/ 0008/78569/001998.pdf**;
- Citizens Advice Bureau *Advice Guide* to patients' rights on **www.adviceguide.org.uk/ index/family_parent/health/nhs_patients_rights.htm#Aboutthisinform ation?**
- Health Rights Information Scotland, *The NHS and You* on **www.hris.org.uk/index. aspx?o=1180**.

Reflect on the following.

- What do these documents assume about healthcare provision and nursing?
- What do they say about the patient?
- Are they reliant on a context or societal expectations?
- Do they define an outcome?
- Do you agree with these documents?

Finally, reflect on these in relation to your personal philosophy for nursing – would you change anything?

Outline answers are given at the end of the chapter.

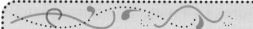

Chapter summary

This chapter has helped you to explore the theoretical principles underpinning nursing as a caring activity and ways in which you might understand the role of the patients, the nurses, the goal of health and the society or environment in which nursing care is given. We have also examined your values and beliefs about giving nursing care and how this can be defined for other people to understand. Critical issues relating to supporting evidence-based practice in nursing today were also explained.

Activities and scenarios: brief outline answers

Case study (Joseph, pages 68–9)

In this case there was no way that Joseph's role as a patient could be self-caring or even negotiating care. As a nurse you had to take control. Now think about what you were actually doing. Your intervention had to take account of the fact that you were on a beach with very limited resources initially. Practically, you needed to make a rapid assessment of Joseph's condition and provide appropriate care and you used a framework or model that you had been taught in order to do this effectively (the ERC guidelines, 2010). The care you had to give needed to change Joseph's internal environment from one that was hypoxic, with an absence of circulation, to one where circulation was effective and breathing allowed gaseous exchange, and this framework enabled this.

Activity 3.6 (page 71)

In examining these documents a picture of nursing and healthcare can be derived that is contextualised within the expectations of contemporary English (UK) healthcare provision. Among other elements you may have identified some of the following:

- the rights of patients and restrictions relating to rights;
- expected behaviours of patients and nurses;
- sense of authority and autonomy and social responsibility for nurses and patients indicating role expectations;
- nursing defined by resource availability and limitations.

You may also have formed opinions about the possibilities of healthcare in the UK, which could shape the way you will plan and deliver care.

Further reading

McKenna, HP and Slevin, O (2008) *Vital Notes for Nurses: Nursing models, theories and practice.* Chichester: Wiley-Blackwell.

This book takes you further in considering the use and application of theoretical perspectives in your nursing practice. It enables you to think about contemporary nursing and the position of theory today.

Tones, K and Green, J (2004) *Health Promotion: Planning and strategies.* New York: Sage.

This book addresses theoretical and practical aspects of planning care for health promotion. It will enable you to develop your thinking about the concept of health in respect of nursing, and how nurses and others can use theoretical perspectives to promote and enhance the health of clients and communities.

Useful websites

www.erc.edu

Although designed primarily for a wide audience, including qualified professionals and educators, this website offers up-to-date advice from the European Resuscitation Council for resuscitation in respiratory and cardiac arrest of adults and children. The algorithm diagrams are useful for those learning the procedures and the sections on end-of-life decisions offer insight.

www.nursingtheory.net/gt_alm.html

This website has helpful summaries of most theories/models and useful links to some theorists' websites.

Chapter 4
The nursing process

Dawn Ritchie

NMC Standards for Pre-registration Nursing Education

This chapter will address the following competencies:

Domain 1: Professional values

3. All nurses must practise with confidence according to The Code: Standards of conduct, performance and ethics for nurses and midwives (NMC 2008a), and within other recognised ethical and legal frameworks. They must be able to recognise and address ethical challenges relating to people's choices and decision making about their care, and act within the law to help them and their families and carers find acceptable solutions.

4. All nurses must practise in a holistic, non-judgemental, caring and sensitive manner that avoids assumptions, supports social inclusion; recognises and respects individual choice; and acknowledges diversity. Where necessary, they must challenge inequality, discrimination and exclusion from access to care.

Domain 2: Communication and interpersonal skills

6. All nurses must use therapeutic principles to engage, maintain and, where appropriate, disengage from professional caring relationships, and must always respect professional boundaries.

Domain 3: Nursing practice and decision making

7. All nurses must practise safely by being aware of the correct use, limitations and hazards of common interventions, including nursing activities, treatments, and the use of medical devices and equipment. The nurse must be able to evaluate their use, report any concerns promptly through appropriate channels and modify care where necessary to maintain safety. They must contribute to the collection of local and national data and formulation of policy on risks, hazards and adverse outcomes.

Domain 4: Leadership, management and team working

5. All nurses must be self-aware and recognise how their own values, principles and assumptions may affect their practice. They must maintain their own personal and professional development, learning from experience, through supervision, feedback, reflection and evaluation.

continued overleaf . . .

continued . . . •••

7. All nurses must work effectively across professional and agency boundaries, actively involving and respecting others' contributions to integrated person-centred care. They must know when and how to communicate with and refer to other professionals and agencies in order to respect the choices of service users and others, promoting shared decision making, to deliver positive outcomes and to coordinate smooth, effective transition within and between services and agencies.

Chapter aims

After reading this chapter, you will be able to:

*   discuss the nursing process as a tool for implementing nursing care;
*   recognise the importance of acknowledging the limitations of your own capabilities;
*   understand your role in ensuring consent, confidentiality and data protection;
*   begin to understand the importance of delivering evidence-based practice.

Introduction

You have now learnt about your role as a nurse professionally, historically and legally, and in terms of the major components of what nurses do and why. Now is the time to put all of this together in practice. This chapter is important for you, because it explores the tools that you need to make nursing work.

In the previous chapter you created a blueprint of a vehicle, identifying all the major features and how they fitted together in your drawings. You were then guided to think about all the major features of nursing and how they fit together. In conclusion, we noted that these were fine on paper but would be no use in practice unless there was a skilled person (a mechanic for the car, or a 'nurse' for nursing), with the appropriate tools to create the actual product (in nursing, the 'healthy' person).

This chapter will look at the tools you will need to nurse effectively in detail. You will be guided to exercises that will make you think about how to use these tools most effectively in practice.

The process of nursing: tools of the trade

Tools are utilised within nursing for a number of reasons, including allowing work to be organised effectively and as a means of documenting care. Tools can also be seen to be educational, since they allow nurses to consider what they are doing for patients and also enable nurses potentially to measure the outcome of care. In addition, they provide a distinct perspective of the discipline that is nursing and act as a foundation on which claims of professional status for nursing rest (as discussed in Chapter 2). By questioning and evaluating practice, nurses are able to generate nursing knowledge that is evidence-based, rather than continuing to do things because 'that is the way they have always been done'.

Possibly the most recognised and widely utilised tool worldwide is the 'nursing process'. This was developed in the USA in the 1960s and introduced to the UK during the 1970s and 1980s. It afforded nurses an opportunity to move away from the more traditional medical model of care delivery, whereby care was divided into a series of tasks undertaken by a number of different nurses, according to levels of experience and skill, and where decision making was carried out by medical staff. The nursing process offers a patient-centred, systematic approach to planning and delivering nursing care using a problem-solving cycle in which the needs of the individual patient are taken into account. It consists of at least four stages.

1. **Assessment**   collecting and considering information from a person or about a person.
2. **Planning**   identifying the nursing care to be delivered to meet that individual's needs through the development of nursing care plans.
3. **Implementation**   carrying out and documenting the nursing care delivered.
4. **Evaluation**   considering whether care that has been delivered has met the needs of the individual.

These four stages are not necessarily separate and sequential steps, and they can take place simultaneously, as will be discussed later. It is important to recognise that the way this tool is used does vary both within and across countries. The adaptation of the nursing process in the UK has been mainly limited to a concentration on the assessment of needs, which is integral to the care process. Some differences do occur internationally, however. For example, in North America the stages are further differentiated with 'nursing diagnoses' being incorporated following the assessment stage and 'defining problems and resources' following the planning stage. Undoubtedly, the problem-solving approach of the nursing process can be seen to be associated with other data-collection processes, such as the research process, whereby the gathering data and subsequent analysis of the information is essential.

Carrying out the nursing process ensures that the nurse considers the whole patient, rather than just the disease or condition to be treated. A central feature of the nursing process is that goals are set according to patients' needs and documented within a nursing care plan, and the extent to which they have been achieved over a specified period of time is considered.

Alternative problem-orientated assessment tools include SOAP, SOAPIE or SOAPIER (using different components of the items in the concept summary below), whereby the nurse identifies and documents the patient's problems. These can be selected according to personal or institutional preferences.

> ### Concept summary: SOAPIER assessment tool
>
> **S** – **S**ubjective data – what the patient, family member or significant other says about what the patient feels or is doing only as relevant to the specific episode of care or problem.
>
> **O** – **O**bjective data – what the healthcare professional observes and tests (in a reproducible manner, such as temperature, pulse, blood pressure, blood glucose, urinalysis, etc).
>
> **A** – **A**ssessment – the nurse's interpretation and professional judgement of both the objective and subjective data in order to justify goals.
>
> **P** – **P**lans – goals, actions, interventions planned.
>
> **I** – **I**mplementation of plan.
>
> **E** – **E**valuates the outcomes of care.
>
> **R** – **R**evision – reconsideration and amendment of the plan if necessary.

Assessment

Assessment is a fundamental skill for all nurses, regardless of field or setting, and is considered to be the first step in providing individualised care. Making assessments or judgements against certain criteria is something undertaken in all aspects of everyday life.

> ### Activity 4.1   *Reflection*
>
> Consider the factors that enable you to determine by what means of transport and also via which route you travel to town for a night out.
>
> You may have considered whether or not you are travelling alone or with friends, distance to be travelled, public transport available, costs involved, whether you are planning to consume alcohol, what time you are planning to return home, local weather conditions, etc.
>
> All of these could be said to be decisive factors in weighing up and deciding on your plans.
>
> *As this activity is based on your own reflection, there is no outline answer at the end of the chapter.*

A nursing assessment involves the comprehensive collation of information about physiological functioning, psychosocial aspects, including family relationships, social networks, educational and/or occupational activities, ethnicity and religious beliefs, and psychological aspects, including, for example, coping strategies, adherence and the patient's conceptualisation of illness.

Assessment strategies in nursing have been influenced by the nursing process, assessment being the first stage.

Activity 4.2   *Critical thinking*

As you will be aware, a number of different nursing assessment proformas are used in clinical practice. They frequently vary between wards within the same NHS Trust, as well as between different fields of nursing.

- Have a look at blank nursing assessment documentation for your own clinical area.
- Identify the framework that underpins nursing assessment in your own area and consider how well the framework was reflected in the organisation of the documentation.

Is there anything that you would like to alter about the documentation in order to improve the assessment process?

As this activity is based on your own observations and reflection, there is no outline answer at the end of the chapter.

Who assesses?

A nursing assessment should be carried out by, or under the supervision of, a 'Named Nurse' with the agreement and cooperation of the patient. A novice nurse will be working under the auspices of a registered nurse who will provide expert support as to what information needs to be obtained in accordance with their professional accountability and responsibility. However, as a student you must at all times act in accordance with the NMC *Code* (2008a) and the NMC *Record Keeping: Guidance for nurses and midwives* (2009c), as well as adhering to national and local NHS Trust policy and guidelines.

It is also important to recognise that nurses do not work in isolation and are frequently working collaboratively with other health and social care professionals, developing and employing integrated assessments such as the Single Assessment Process (SAP) for Older People (DH, 2002b). These collaborative tools are important in providing a more efficient assessment process; however, it is important to recognise that they do not make a nursing assessment redundant. The intention is to avoid unnecessary duplication by sharing information and utilising resources effectively with the different health and social care professionals contributing to the assessment process in the most effective way.

A nursing assessment is generally undertaken when a nurse first meets a patient, regardless of the setting. This could be within a community situation, or visiting a patient in their home or at a health centre, during an outpatient clinic appointment, or within a more acute setting, including on admission to hospital or on transfer to different clinical areas, such as critical care areas. The term 'assessment' can imply that this is a once-only process, whereas 'assessing' would perhaps be a more accurate description of what nurses do, since the process should be ongoing and dependent upon whether there is an improvement or deterioration in the patient. Assessing or reassessment is usually undertaken as part of each interaction with clients.

Assessment information is collected primarily from the patient themselves or, if they are not able to participate in this process either temporarily or permanently (due to mental incapacity as a result of sedatory effects of medications, or a loss of consciousness or coma, or mental illness, or being, in the case of minors, developmentally inappropriate), information about the patient may be obtained from secondary sources. These secondary sources include family, significant others such as friends or carers, and through reviewing already accumulated information within patient records/nursing notes and from other health and social care professionals involved with the patient. It is vital to consider that not all information is required immediately at the initial assessment, and assessment is generally ongoing with information being gathered over a period of time. Judgement is required to prioritise essential initial assessment data. The ability of nurses to use information and make decisions about care needs and delivery is more effective the more expert they become.

Consent and confidentiality

To be able to attain personal and private information from another person requires the development of a trusting relationship and consent must be gained for both the collection of information and the use of it. It is the nurse's responsibility to provide the patient with enough information, using language that the patient understands, so that the patient will have sufficient knowledge to understand why nursing assessment will assist in their care delivery and management. If there are concerns regarding the patient's understanding, which, for example, may be the result of language difficulties, additional assistance such as the use of interpreters must be sought.

In nursing assessment, patients may often be expected to disclose confidential and frequently sensitive information before a relationship has had an opportunity to become fully established. It is, therefore, imperative that the patient who is in the care of a nurse believes that any information given is treated as confidential.

Activity 4.3   *Critical thinking*

You may find it beneficial to look at the NMC advice sheet on confidentiality, accessible at **www.nmc-uk.org/Nurses-and-midwives/Advice-by-topic/A/Advice/confidentiality**

- In what circumstances could a nurse be reasonably expected to disclose confidential information without consent?
- Identify specific examples when disclosure without consent may occur within different clinical settings.
- What special considerations need to be taken into account when disclosure is being considered?

Outline answers are given at the end of the chapter.

All nurses are professionally accountable and as a student the same principles of confidentiality apply. It is the responsibility of the individual to follow local procedures for handling and storing information. Any information obtained must be kept in accordance with both the NMC *Code*

(2007a) and the Data Protection Act (2000). Access to health records is restricted according to the Access to Health Records Act (1990), the Data Protection Act (2000), the Freedom of Information Act (2000) and Freedom of Information (Scotland) Act (2002). (Visit **www.opsi.gov.uk** for details of all these acts.)

Concept summary: The Data Protection Act

The Data Protection Act (2000) aims to protect the rights and interests of individuals by stringently regulating the storage and use of information, whether held on paper or on computer. It also gives rights to individuals to know what information is held about them.

Further information can be obtained from:

* **www.ico.gov.uk/Home/for_the_public/topic_specific_guides/health.aspx;**
* **www.ico.gov.uk/upload/documents/library/data_protection/detailed_ specialist_guides/how_does_the_data_protection_act_apply_to_professional_ opinions.pdf.**

Within the assessment process there is both a legal and professional duty to provide a fully documented account of the assessment and the care that has subsequently been planned and delivered.

The patient assessment

If assessment is to be meaningful, it must be individualised and comprehensive. Nursing assessment seeks to provide an accurate picture of the patient's current condition, compared to medical diagnosis, which aims to provide a causal explanation for the patient's presenting signs and symptoms. The early recognition of potential and actual factors affecting the patient, accompanied by an appropriate response, is achieved by the collation of data through both observation and interview.

Observation

Observation is something undertaken by humans continuously, and is frequently a subconscious activity. Consider for a moment the number of times you see or hear things that you do not register. How often do you hear someone say 'I didn't see that', or recognise that, although you may have been appearing to listen to someone, you have no recollection of what they have been saying.

In nursing, it is important that such observation is noticed and included within the patient assessment. Further, while in everyday life there is generally no requirement to retain or record observations and this information can be discarded, in nursing this information must be carefully documented.

There are two types of observational data – objective and subjective.

> ## Concept summary: Objective and subjective data
>
> **Objective data** – includes those observations that can be measured, such as fundamental nursing observations or vital signs, including pulse, respiratory rate, blood pressure, temperature and weight.
>
> **Subjective data** – includes how an individual interacts, non-verbal communication and reaction to their surroundings. It may also include how they don't react. For example, a person who has sustained a head injury may not recognise relatives.

Systematic observation

Observation skills are not innate and, therefore, there are a number of challenges if clinical observational skills are going to be used effectively. Nurses need to learn to watch and listen not only attentively, but also systematically. This is where an assessment framework based on a nursing model, such as Roper et al.'s Activities of Living (1983; 2000), can be utilised to provide a systematic approach so that nothing is missed.

The importance of including the individual within the assessment process cannot be over-emphasised and patients should usually be regarded as equal partners in the compilation of their records. The patients' subjective interpretation of how they are feeling, what they describe their symptoms to be and what they perceive to be happening informs the process. Such holistic assessment requires time in order to establish a relationship with individual patients, so that they are able to provide honest and open responses to potentially sensitive questions. Therefore, it is imperative that the nurse undertaking the assessment has effective verbal and non-verbal communication skills. If the person being assessed is unable to contribute, for example as a result of mental incapacity, family members', significant others' or carers' understanding of experiences should be taken into account. Collaboration with others is essential. For example, it is recognised in the paediatric setting that parents are excellent in identifying indicators of their children's illnesses.

The initial patient interview will require the collection of biographical information, such as name, date of birth, sex, home address (usual place of residence) and next of kin. It is essential that accurate information is detailed to avoid identification errors and also to prevent offence, particularly given the varying cultural norms for recording first and family names.

The majority of NHS Trusts require an individual to formally nominate a next of kin on admission. Next of kin can be a family member, partner or close friend. While they are unable to consent to or refuse treatment on an individual's behalf, they can offer opinions to inform decision making if the individual is unable to do so. The age of an individual is relevant, so that care can be managed by appropriate personnel and departments, and be referred in order to access relevant support services. In addition, when a child or young person is admitted to hospital, the person(s) with parental responsibility needs to be identified.

Concept summary: Parental responsibility

Parental responsibility is defined in section 3(1) of the Children Act 1989 as being:

all the rights, duties, powers, responsibilities and authority which by law a parent of a child has in relation to the child and his property.
(HM Government, 1989)

The term 'parental responsibility' attempts to focus on the parents' duties towards their child rather than the parents' rights over their child. Parental responsibility includes the right of parents to consent to treatment on behalf of their child provided it is in the child's best interest.

Further clarification on parental responsibility can be obtained at: **www.bma.org. uk/ethics/consent_and_capacity/Parental.jsp**.

Further information might include past and current medical history, growth and development, family relationships, occupation or school, housing or living accommodation, and religious beliefs. These are important in providing a comprehensive assessment for holistic care.

Acquiring and interpreting assessment information is dependent upon the knowledge, ability and skill of the nurse in communicating and building relationships effectively. The nurse must also be able to interpret the information received appropriately in order to develop a plan of care. For this reason, the overall nursing assessment is usually linked to a framework for health assessment, so that the quality of assessment is enhanced.

Nolan and Caldock (1996) suggest that any framework for assessment should be:

*   flexible and able to be adapted to a variety of circumstances;
*   appropriate to the audience it is intended for;
*   capable of balancing and incorporating the views of carers, users and agencies;
*   able to provide a mechanism for bringing different views together, while recognising the diversity and variation within individual circumstances.

A number of nursing assessment tools are available but probably the most familiar tool in the United Kingdom is Roper et al.'s (1983; 2000) Activities of Living Model. According to this model, one of the best ways to understand and thereby identify and articulate the needs of an individual is in relation to the 12 activities of living. Roper et al. identified these as:

1. maintaining a safe environment;
2. communicating;
3. breathing;

4. eating and drinking;

5. eliminating;

6. personal cleansing and dressing;

7. controlling body temperature;

8. mobilising;

9. working and playing;

10. expressing sexuality;

11. sleeping;

12. dying.

Each of these activities of living is seen to have five dimensions – physical, physiological, socio-cultural, environmental and politico-economic.

Activity 4.4   *Reflection*

In relation to mobilising, which is identified within the activities of living, think about what activities you have undertaken today that require the use of both arms. Now imagine that you have fallen down the stairs and broken your dominant arm.

Reflect upon how this would impact upon your mobility.

- Which of the activities identified above would you no longer be able to undertake?
- Which activities would you require assistance to be able to undertake safely?

As this activity is based on your own reflection, there is no outline answer at the end of the chapter.

Just as in the activity above, at assessment the nurse aims to establish what the patient can or cannot do in each of the activities of living. The nurse does need to take into account the individual's dependence/independence, which will vary according to age, developmental capabilities, circumstances and environment. A nine-month-old infant will be wholly dependent upon parents or carers, whereas a 44-year-old lady diagnosed with multiple sclerosis may be independent in a number of activities but may require assistance with elimination and mobilising.

Assessment within assessment

Using a framework such as Roper et al.'s Activities of Living Model (1983; 2000) facilitates the systematic collection of information about essential care components. However, it is also important to recognise that this is only the first step in providing information relating to the general care needs of the individual. A number of specific assessment tools have been developed to attain measurable outcomes, since these provide more objective measurements and reduce subjectivity inherent in either patients' descriptions or nurses' observations. These include assessment tools such as pressure sore risk calculators, for example the Norton and Waterlow assessment tools, moving and handling assessment tools, nutritional assessment tools, pain assessment tools, anxiety and depression scales and the Glasgow Coma Scale.

The Waterlow Score

All patients admitted to hospital must have their risk of developing a pressure sore assessed and documented within six hours of admission (NICE/RCN, 2005). The Waterlow Score is possibly the most widely used pressure risk assessment tool in the UK and is used in both community and acute care settings across all age groups. It is a relatively simplistic tool that is easily applied and assesses a patient's risk of developing pressure ulcers by quantifying a range of commonly acknowledged risk factors, including sex, age, skin type, mobility, continence, nutritional status, etc. This is essential in identifying patients at risk and in ensuring that the right interventions or treatment modalities are able to be applied appropriately. Using the Waterlow Score takes a matter of minutes, but it needs to be used in conjunction with clinical judgement. It is not a one-off assessment and reassessments should be undertaken throughout a patient's care.

The Glasgow Coma Scale

The Glasgow Coma Scale (GCS) is used to assess and quantify levels of consciousness. It is relatively quick, accurate and simple, and can be used in patients of all ages, provided an age-adapted tool such as James and Trauner's adaptation (1985) is used for infants and children.

The level of consciousness is a sensitive and objective indicator of neurological functioning. Consciousness is assessed by measuring the best response of three components:

- eye opening;
- verbal response;
- motor response.

Each component has a scoring scale describing levels of responsiveness. Summation of the score of each component ranges from 3 to 15. A score of 15 indicates full consciousness, whereas a score of 8 or less indicates coma.

As indicated above, the score becomes lower as the degree of neurological impairment increases. The GCS has been the subject of numerous studies to test reliability and has been found to be used reliably and accurately by experienced and highly trained users. However, inexperienced users are identified as making consistent errors, particularly in patients who are at intermediate levels of consciousness, that is, they are neither fully conscious with a score of 15, nor comatose with a score of 8 or less. This does call into question its use by inexperienced staff without adequate supervision.

The Hospital Anxiety and Depression Scale

The Hospital Anxiety and Depression Scale is a commonly used, self-rating questionnaire used to screen for mild degrees of mood disorder, anxiety and depression. It was originally designed for use in the outpatient setting and is extensively used in primary care. It consists of 14 questions – seven for anxiety and seven for depression. Patients are asked to identify the reply that comes closest to describing how they have been feeling over the past week. Patients do need to record their immediate response as it does tend to be a more accurate indicator than a long and thought-out response.

The specific measurement instruments discussed above are examples of instruments that can be used to inform and support nursing assessment, but numerous other tools are available. What is common with these tools is that all have been validated following extensive reliability testing. Likewise, they are all relatively quick and simple to apply in practice and allow for the collection over time of comparable data. This capacity for reproduction reinforces the ongoing nature of assessment.

Making sense of information gained during the assessment process is vital to ensure accurate identification of the patient's problems. Throughout the assessment process a review of data will have been ongoing, with decisions being made as to the meaning and significance of information obtained. Consideration will be given as to whether there are any variances in the information the patient has provided and what the nurse has observed. For example, a patient may state that they are not in any pain and yet the nurse, through observation, may identify that there are behavioural and physiological indices of pain. The patient may be pale, clammy, grimacing, reluctant to move, tachycardic and hypertensive, all of which are indices of pain. The real significance of this information needs to be interpreted in light of other information the nurse needs to elicit. In the above situation the nurse, through further questioning and clarification, may establish that the patient's reluctance to acknowledge their pain is due to a previous bad experience of pain, and fear of having an injection administered to control the pain, since they are needle phobic. Judgements about the quantity and quality of information require considerable skill. Experienced nurses are able to handle large volumes of information, and quickly and easily establish the interrelationship between them. For novice nurses the links between separate pieces of information are not always easy to establish and, as knowledge and understanding increase, so will the capacity to analyse information.

By analysing and establishing the significance of the information obtained, the nurse is attempting to establish whether any aspect of the activities of living is problematic or potentially problematic for that individual patient. There has been considerable debate about the use of the term 'problem', but Roper et al. (1983; 2000) do endorse its use within their model of nursing, since they describe nursing as helping patients to solve, alleviate or cope with or prevent problems with their activities of living. It is vital when identifying problems to remember that they are the patient's problems and need to be focused on the patient. Potential problems relate to something that may occur, for example the identification that the patient is at risk of developing a pressure sore, after you have undertaken a risk assessment utilising the Waterlow Score. It is also important to acknowledge that, in a number of areas, a multidisciplinary approach to assessment and problem identification has been adopted. Increasingly, common documentation frameworks are being used to avoid patients being subject to repetitious assessments by health and social care professionals, and in order to improve the quality and efficiency of care.

Assessment can appear simple and, as a consequence, can be undervalued, and yet it is a fundamental and necessarily complex process for the delivery of effective care.

Care priorities

The prioritising of care need is a central part of the nursing process. Prioritising care follows patient assessment and diagnosis, and is the process of determining needs and goals. Planning then aims to develop a course of action aimed at meeting the patient's needs and meeting the prioritised goals of care.

Developing goals

Goals derive from patient problems, both actual and potential, identified within the assessment stage. Goal setting according to Leach (2008, p1729) *assists both the client and practitioner in identifying and prioritising strategies that may prevent, reduce or resolve client problems, or that facilitate or augment client function.* Goals must be prioritised, with those that are life-threatening or pose the highest level of risk to the patient being given the highest priority.

Goals can be immediate, for example resuscitating a patient brought into the Emergency Department following a road traffic accident; short term, for example for a patient with a dependence upon alcohol to abstain from having a drink for a week; or long term, for example a client with learning disability developing an understanding and an ability to communicate using alternative means, such as Makaton or PECS (picture exchange communication system). Goals imply a future desirable outcome and are sometimes referred to the final point that the patient is expected to reach.

Creating goals improves organisational efficiency and enhances patient care, but it is not an innate process; the majority of patients have complex situations that require professional knowledge and understanding in order for goals to be planned in a realistic, systematic and patient-centred manner. In order to achieve this, Wright (2005) suggests that goals should be SMART: specific, measurable, agreed, realistic and time limited.

Concept summary: SMART

Specific – goals need to be very clear and unambiguous. Both the patient and nurse should be able to specify what they expect to achieve.

Measurable – goals need to be able to be measured either directly or indirectly, since it is vital that an improvement or deterioration can be detected or measured.

Achievable – goals need to ensure that you have the resources available to achieve them. This is sometimes substituted with the word 'agreed', which is a helpful adjunct when working with patients.

Realistic – one of the most frequent complaints about care plans is that they are unrealistic and, therefore, it is imperative that small incremental goals are set.

Time limited – all goals should have a time limit by which they should be achieved. This means that goals need to be reviewed on a regular basis, so that the partners involved can agree whether or not the goal has been achieved. Review meetings do need to be flexible, since some goals may be achieved more rapidly, whereas others may require refinement.

Leach (2008) identifies a number of key elements required for effective goal setting.

- The client should be actively involved.
- Goals should be clear and specific.
- Goals should be measurable.
- The cost of treatment should be taken into consideration.

Goals should also be clear and specific so that both patients and practitioners understand what is intended. Think about the number of times you may have been told to 'keep an eye' on something. What precisely does this mean if you are escorting a client with a learning disability on a shopping trip? Or if you are asked to keep an eye on a young person with suicidal thoughts? Or if you are asked to keep an eye on an intravenous infusion? To know what to do requires some knowledge and a plan of action. The care plan, therefore, needs to be clear and specific enough to prevent anybody getting the wrong impression about what is happening and to remove any confusion.

Developing goals should be a collaborative process that empowers individuals to take control of their health. It is particularly important that clients are involved in developing mutually agreed goals, since their cooperation, understanding and motivation are vital if goals are to be realised. In addition, there is also the ethical issue of the patient's right to be involved in decisions about their own health.

A more traditional paternalistic approach is seen also. In this approach, healthcare professionals do not engage patients in the planning process but still anticipate their compliance. It is, however, naive to assume that patients' and professionals' goals will always be the same, especially when professional opinions do not always concur! The rationales given for staff failing to actively involve patients include a lack of time, perceived lack of ability of the individual, and lack of ability of staff.

Leach (2008) proposes that a two-stage process is undertaken in order to effectively plan care.

1. The construction of a general overall, desired outcome of care. This broad goal would not specifically state how the goal would be achieved.
2. The creation of an expected outcome or specific goal. This specifies how and by when the patient will achieve the goal.

Leach (2008, p1732) identifies a number of questions to assist patients and practitioners in identifying appropriate treatment goals.

Overall concerns

1a. What are your main health concerns at present?
1b. Which of these issues concerns you the most? Why?
1c. How does this health concern affect you – physically, socially, emotionally and financially?
1d. How would you like to see this health concern improve over the next few days or months?

(Questions 1c and 1d can be asked to explore each of the issues raised in question 1a.)

Presenting condition

2a. In relation to your presenting condition, what is your main concern? Why?

2b. How does this health concern affect you – physically, socially, emotionally and financially?

2c. How would you like to see this health concern improve in the short term and in the long term?

Care planning

The purpose of the nursing care plan is to have an easily accessible document that details the planned nursing interventions not only to the nursing staff, but also to the patient and relatives. Each care plan should be unique to the individual patient and is composed of a set of problems derived from the assessment and the associated interventions required to address that patient's needs. The person who is responsible for ensuring the actions to be taken to enable achievement of the goals is the registered nurse allocated to care for the patient. The care plan also forms part of the patient's permanent care record.

Care planning should be a dynamic and evolving process. It must enable the actual intervention and evaluation of care and, therefore, it is critical to ensure that it is realistic and sensitive to patient need, as well as designed to achieve the prioritised goals of care. In order to be effective, care planning also needs to be delivered on an individualised basis using a structured framework. In some situations (for example, emergency or short-stay settings), an initial brief or 'short' care plan may be developed or required after a rapid initial assessment. This will entail identifying needs, setting goals and planning interventions to meet initial needs.

This initial care plan can be focused on specific needs and then, as a relationship is able to be developed over a period of time, a more comprehensive assessment may be undertaken.

Figure 4.1 is an example of what a care plan may look like.

In conclusion, care planning is not an inherent skill; however, the process can be facilitated by following a systematic approach and basing it on reason. Care plans do need to be clear and, even if patients have wide-ranging needs, care plans should not be complex. They need to be client-centred and expected outcomes need to be mutually agreed, specific, measurable, achievable, realistic and time limited (SMART). Care planning ought to be a transparent process, which, as part of quality assurance, should be subject to scrutiny through audit at a local level. This can assist in identifying if services are client-focused, the range of interventions required, which agencies may be involved in care, and any gaps in communication and collaboration of care, as well as assist in informing staff development and training needs.

Implementation

The implementation of a care plan is a distinctive stage within the nursing process and, as such, creates different challenges to those identified within both the assessment and planning stages. There are a number of definitions of implementation within the literature, but within this context implementation fundamentally means putting the plan of nursing care into action.

Factors influencing the implementation of nursing activities include not only the quality of the assessment and planning stage, but also the care delivery system used and resources available.

Date:	*Problem number*:	*Patient identity details*:

Problem: Joe has abdominal pain

Goal: Joe will experience no pain or a reduced level of pain acceptable to him

Nursing interventions/*rationales*

- Assess and record Joe's pain through the use of questioning, including type and location of pain, how long it lasts, whether it travels – *to enable accurate assessment of pain.*

- Assess and record pain using a pain assessment tool, such as a visual analogue scale 0–10 for adults (with 0 being no pain and 10 being extreme pain) or Wong–Baker FACES pain-rating scale for children – *in order to attempt to identify how bad the pain is.*

- Evaluate Joe's status by observing his behaviour and vital signs – *in order to assess for behavioural indices of pain, such as grimacing, diaphoresis (sweating), pallor and alterations in vital signs, including increased pulse, respiratory rate and elevated BP.*

- Administer analgesics as prescribed and as required – *for pain relief.*

- Use non-pharmacologic methods of pain relief, such as distraction therapy, imagery, self-hypnosis – *non-pharmacological pain management is the management of pain without medications; this method utilises ways to alter thoughts and focus concentration to better manage and reduce pain.*

- Monitor and document the effectiveness of analgesics and/or non-pharmacological interventions – *in order to ensure that Joe is receiving and has been prescribed adequate analgesics and/or the non-pharmacological interventions are effective.*

- Involve clinical pain nurse specialist in Joe's care – *can provide expert knowledge and support to nursing and medical staff.*

- Discuss all care and treatment with Joe – *to minimise anxiety and distress, and enable his full participation in care and treatment.*

Nursing evaluation:
Date:
Evaluation of nursing interventions:
Sign and print name and designation:

Figure 4.1: Sample care plan

Consideration needs to be given as to how the interventions documented within the care plan are translated into care delivered to the patient.

Evidence-based practice

A central tenet of the NMC *Code* (2008a) is a requirement for nurses' knowledge and skills to be kept up to date and, as a student participating in care delivery, you likewise must deliver care based on the best available evidence or best practice. This can be extremely challenging, since nursing practice is constantly evolving. There are a number of resources available to assist you in implementing best practice. In all clinical areas there should be local policies and procedures accessible to staff. The purpose of a policy is to provide a framework of principles outlining the responsibilities of staff in ensuring the effective management of a course of action. Policies may reflect statutory requirements.

Activity 4.5   *Research and evidence-based practice*

In your practice learning experience find your local NHS Trust policy for the administration of medications. Consider the following questions.

- Where was evidence of the local policy located? Was it easily accessible? What are the implications for care delivery if you had difficulty locating the policy?
- Is any reference made to any statutory requirements?
- What evidence is there that the policy has been based upon best available evidence/best practice?
- Does the policy have a time-frame for being updated or reviewed? Why is this important?

As this activity is based on your own reflection, there is no outline answer at the end of the chapter.

Some of the most widely used terms within nursing today are evidence-based nursing and evidence-based practice, and there are many definitions available as to what evidence-based practice encompasses. DiCenso and Cullum (1998, p38) state: *Evidence-based nursing integrates the best evidence from research with clinical expertise, patient preferences, and existing resources into decision making about the health care of individual patients*. It is apparent from this definition that evidence-based nursing requires nurses to make decisions about what is best evidence and how this can be used in the best interests of individual patients within the resources available. It is not possible within the current climate to make decisions about healthcare based solely on the clinical effectiveness of an intervention. Consideration must also be given to the resource implications, with cost being a major factor in the decision-making equation. So, although evidence-based healthcare is used to enhance the care of individuals, it can be and is also used to inform wider policy decisions to improve the health of the population as a whole. This can, on occasions, lead to a variance as to what is in the best interests of the public as a whole versus those of an individual.

Asking questions

Evidence-based healthcare starts with having an enquiring mind, asking questions and recognising issues that you would like to explore further. It is about recognising that there are multiple perspectives for understanding and analysing things, and also looking for solutions. In order to act in a manner that is based on evidence, 'the nurse needs to knit together many sources of evidence' (Ellis, 2011, p5). It is imperative that you question the actions of both yourself and others when delivering care. The most frequent questions within practice relate directly to the care of patients and are frequently prefaced with 'Why do we do this?', 'What would happen if . . .?', 'How can we improve this?' and 'When is the best time to . . .?'

Asking questions is in itself not sufficient, being only the first part of the evidence-based practice process. The next stage is to find the evidence, and this is becoming a more complex process as our ability to access information increases and the volume of nursing and health-related literature rapidly expands. The majority of people gain information on an ad hoc basis, either from browsing through books and journals, or by seeing and hearing information within the media. There is a very real danger of being overwhelmed when first looking for evidence and, in order to focus your reading, Crombie suggests the following steps.

- Clarify your reasons for reading – develop your question or hypothesis.
- Specify the information required – identify the keywords in relation to your question and decide where you are going to look for evidence, e.g. electronic databases such as CINAHL, Medline, Cochrane or through organisations such as National Institute for Health and Clinical Excellence (NICE).
- Identify the relevant reports –reject any unhelpful material.
- Critically appraise the paper.

(Crombie, 2007, p1)

Sources of information

Cochrane Collaboration – cochrane.co.uk/ – produces and disseminates systematic reviews of healthcare interventions.

National Institute for Health and Clinical Excellence (NICE) – www.nice.org.uk – an independent organisation that produces national guidance in three areas: public health, health technologies and clinical practice.

The Centre for Evidence Based Medicine – www.cebm.net – has some useful tools that can assist you in the development of critical appraisal skills, including asking focused questions, finding evidence, levels of evidence, searching evidence, critical appraisal, making a decision and evaluating performance.

Additional websites that can assist you include:

Critical Appraisal Skills Programme – www.phru.nhs.uk/Pages/PHD/resources. htm – has developed tools to assist in the critical appraisal of articles, including types of research such as:

- systematic reviews;
- randomised controlled trials;
- qualitative research;
- cohort studies; etc.

AGREE Collaboration – www.agreecollaboration.org – assesses the quality of clinical guidelines.

Participating in care delivery

As a student you will participate in implementing care delivery, but this will always be under the supervision of a registered nurse. This supervision initially will be close, with the nurse observing all actions in order to satisfy themselves of your competency, while on other occasions supervision may be at a distance, meaning that the nurse is available for support within the ward area but not directly observing actions undertaken. Students are supernumerary in all placements, but they can and do take on increasing responsibilities as part of the nursing team as they progress through the training programme. Nonetheless, for a student to participate in the care, the registered nurse will first need to establish whether the student is capable of carrying out the instructions given and able to provide care of a required standard.

How the registered nurse determines a student's capability will vary. It can be ascertained by the nurse questioning the student to determine if they have sufficient knowledge and understanding of what is required, or they may ask whether the student has been taught the underpinning theory within the university setting and whether they had an opportunity to practise the skill through simulation, or whether it is something they have undertaken on an earlier learning experience allocation. The registered nurse supervising may decide it is appropriate to teach the student to perform the care activity if it is something that they have not previously encountered. Alternatively, the registered nurse may have seen the student perform the activity previously and already made a decision regarding the student's competence to perform the activity safely. When a nurse delegates care, they retain accountability for the patient and so they must ensure that delegation is appropriate and that the care given has been correct (NMC, 2008a). Consequently, as a student working under the supervision of different registered nurses, either on the same learning experience allocation or when changing placements, each registered nurse will need to assure themselves that you are competent to undertake any aspect of care that they deem is appropriate to be delegated.

Although the registered nurse is accountable to the NMC for care that has been delegated, this does not mean as a pre-registration student that you cannot be held responsible or accountable for your actions or omissions. You can be called to account by your university and/or by the law for your actions or omissions. Therefore, at all times you should only work within your level of knowledge and competence. As a nursing student you are expected to carry out care at a standard deemed 'reasonable' for a nursing student at the same level of knowledge and skills. The courts would judge your actions against what a reasonable student of the same level of education would have done. This is known as the Bolam Test, which, although originally applied to medicine, is now widely accepted for other professional groups, including nursing.

Concept summary: The Bolam Test

The test for the standard of care stems from the well-known medical negligence case of *Bolam v. Friern Hospital Management Committee* (1957) and is generally known as the Bolam Test.

James Bolam had been admitted to the Friern Hospital for electroconvulsive therapy (ECT). This was administered without the use of muscle relaxants and anaesthetic agents. Unfortunately, Mr Bolam fell off the table and sustained a number of fractures. Mr Bolam alleged that the hospital was negligent. The presiding judge ruled that a doctor is not guilty of negligence if he is acting in accordance with practice accepted as proper by a responsible body of doctors exercising that particular skill and, in this case, determined that there was no negligence involved. The standard of care provided is not assessed with the benefit of hindsight, but instead is looked at on the basis of what the medical professional knew or should have known at the time the treatment was provided. One of the key features of the Bolam principle is that it develops as standards of care develop.

Thus, what may have been considered good practice a number of years ago may now lead to a prosecution for negligence.

This is not always as easy as it may first appear, since everyday practice involves complex decisions about working within the limits of your competence and recognising your own limitations. However, as a student it is imperative that you do not participate in any activity for which you have not been fully prepared or in which you are not adequately supervised.

Activity 4.6   *Critical thinking*

As a student you are studying for both a university award and a professional qualification. Consequently, you are expected to comply with both your university and the NMC guidelines regarding conduct.

Locate and read both your university's guidance on conduct and also the NMC *Code* (2008a) accessible via **www.nmc-uk.org**.

Be aware that conduct that is seen to contravene your university's guidance or the *Code* may give rise to concerns regarding your fitness to practise and ultimately may have implications for your NMC registration.

As this activity is based on your own observations, there is no outline answer at the end of the chapter.

Implementation, as stated earlier, is about delivering care and, in order to begin care delivery, as obvious as it may sound, you do need to actually read the care plan and also receive a handover to ensure that you know what is required in order to accomplish each individual patient's goals. The care plan can then be put into action through safe, competent practice.

Success of implementation depends on the initial assessment, quality of the nursing care plan, and organisation of the care delivery and competence of the care given. Frequently, it also entails the support and involvement of multidisciplinary teams and, without an individualised care plan, nursing care can become fragmented.

Evaluation

Post-implementation, the care delivered needs to be considered in order to judge its value, quality and the extent to which it has achieved its intended outcome. Evaluation of care involves reviewing the patient's progress by comparing the actual patient outcomes with the original goal identified during the care planning stage. By consistently, systematically and rigorously evaluating, the quality of care delivered to patients should be enhanced. This is because it enables nurses to understand what works and what does not work.

Evaluation should be an ongoing process, as it enables continuous assessment and planning as individuals' circumstances and problems change. Evaluation needs to concentrate on the outcome measures chosen. It can focus on quantitative assessments of achievement, such as physiological observations of heart rate, blood pressure, respiratory rate, weight, etc., or qualitative approaches focusing on interpretation of more subjective data such as interviews with the patient exploring how a goal has been achieved.

Best practice promotes the involvement of the patient, his or her relatives or carers and other healthcare professionals. By involving the patient, suppositions about the effectiveness of care delivered should be avoided, making evaluation a more objective process.

Phases of evaluation

Evaluation can occur on a continuous, hourly, daily or longer basis depending on the patient's problem and the timescale set for achievement. There are a number of steps that need to be considered when evaluating care. You will need to:

* establish whether the goals have been completely met, partially met, or not met at all;
* consider the accuracy of the prior assessment;
* think about the relative contribution and the duration of the intervention;
* assess whether the timescale for goal achievement was realistic;
* take into account whether any alterations are needed in the care plan;
* record any findings.
    – If the goal has been completely achieved, you will need to document the evidence for achievement and discontinue the care interventions.
    – If the goal has only been partially met or not met at all, you will need to consider why. If the problem needs reassessing or if the plan of care needs modifying, document accordingly.

Questions you may want to ask
* Has progress been made towards attainment of the goal?
* Has the problem deteriorated? (A movement away from the goal)
* Has the problem changed?
* Was the goal appropriate?
* Was the lack of progress due to the way care was implemented?
* Was the nursing care appropriate?
* Is additional information required?
* Was the timescale appropriate?

An integral part of evaluating care is communicating and recording the care process.

The importance of communication in care delivery

Effective communication, both with other team members and across different disciplines of nursing activities, is critical in facilitating high-quality care. The need for information sharing has been recognised as not only making more effective use of resources, thereby allowing staff more time to deliver services, but also as being essential in promoting and safeguarding well-being. Much of the criticism pertaining to recent high-profile child-protection cases, including that concerning Baby Peter, has been levelled at the failure to share information between agencies (Laming, 2009).

Recent Government thinking centres on information sharing and particularly the concepts of openness and transparency in the way that services are delivered. This is happening more and more within health services and is reflected not only in interdisciplinary working, but also with the expansion of the co-location of agencies, for example children's centres.

Record keeping

Record keeping is an integral part of nursing and is considered by the NMC (2010, p1) to be *essential to the provision of safe and effective care. It is not an optional extra to be fitted in if circumstances allow.*

The aim of good record keeping is to ensure that colleagues know what care has been assessed, has been undertaken or is planned for the future, and how care has been evaluated.

Students are required to gain the knowledge and skills they require to record information effectively and accurately on both paper and computer-held records according to both legal and local requirements. As a student, if you are the person carrying out care, you should document what has taken place within the care record, recording the date, time of writing and signature. There is a requirement within the standards of health records established by the NHS Litigation Authority (NHSLA, 2005) for signatures to be clearly and easily identifiable. In addition, when a student completes the care record there is a requirement for it to be countersigned by a registered nurse.

Traditionally, much information has been passed on verbally, for example through the nursing handover or ward round; however, this can result in selective editing of information and a failure to pass on pertinent information.

Standards of record keeping are considered to be a reflection of an individual's level of professional practice. Good record keeping is regarded as reflecting a safe and competent practitioner, whereas poor record keeping is often judged as reflecting concerns and/or shortfalls within that individual's practice. It is vital to remember that, should records be called as evidence within a court case, the legal system tends to adopt the approach that 'if it is not recorded, it has not been done'.

| Activity 4.7 | *Research and evidence-based practice* |

Look up the NMC guidance on record keeping at **www.nmc-uk.org/Documents/ Guidance/nmcGuidanceRecordKeepingGuidanceforNursesandMidwives. pdf**

Having read the NMC guidance on record keeping, write down six errors that commonly occur in healthcare records.

Brief outline answers are given at the end of the chapter.

Evaluation is a dynamic process concerned with the effectiveness of the care delivered. Evaluation skills are similar to assessment skills and include observing, questioning, examining, measuring, recording and reflecting. The effectiveness of evaluation within health services does require practitioners to base their practices upon the best available evidence. As nurses we must be able to justify our actions. We need to know whether what we are doing is right or at least not wrong.

Chapter summary

This chapter has explored the issues concerned with 'doing nursing'. By using a tool such as the nursing process, the value of using a framework to guide care delivery has been established. It was recognised that other tools and models of nursing are also used.

Operational issues of assessing, planning, implementing and evaluating care have been explored. It was recognised that the patient is nowadays expected to participate more fully in their treatment and care, and emphasis has been placed upon providing patients with adequate information to do so. You have been introduced to some of the issues that pose challenges to the delivery of effective care, including confidentiality, consent, record keeping and evidence-based practice, and you have been asked to consider critically your own practice.

Through a greater understanding of the nursing process, you will be able to develop a sense of how to nurse effectively and understand more clearly the knowledge, skills and values that a nurse contributes.

Activities: brief outline answers

Activity 4.3 (page 78)

Nurses could be reasonably expected to disclose confidential information without consent only in exceptional circumstances when they believe that someone may be at risk of harm. Nurses must always act in accordance within the law of the country where they are practising.

Examples of times when disclosure without consent may occur include situations such as:

- child protection;
- when dealing with domestic violence – child protection issues must override the normal confidentiality and data protection considerations;
- when dealing with parents or carers with a mental health illness – child protection issues must override the normal confidentiality and data protection considerations;
- injuries sustained from knife wounds or gunshot wounds;
- providing the police, when asked, with the name and address of drivers who are allegedly guilty of an offence contrary to the Road Traffic Act (1998);
- dealing with notifiable diseases as required under the Public Health (Infectious Diseases) 1988 Act and the Public Health (Control of Diseases) 1988 Act.

As a student, it is good practice always to discuss a decision to disclose information with senior professional colleagues and, if appropriate, professional bodies such as the RCN.

If an exceptional decision to disclose is made, the nurse making that decision must be able to justify their actions. Therefore, it is imperative that a clear and accurate account is recorded in the patient's records, dated, timed and signed. In some circumstances it may not be appropriate to inform the person of the decision to disclose. For example, if there is a threat of a violent response.

The Data Protection Act (1998) does allow in very rare circumstances for health care professionals to restrict access to information which they hold on a person in their care, if that information is likely to cause harm to the individual or another person. A decision to store information in a supplementary record should only be made in exceptional circumstances, the reason for this must be able to be justified and all members of the healthcare team should be aware of this record. Any information contained within this supplementary record is subject to the same requirements of record keeping and should not compromise the person's confidentiality.

Activity 4.7 (page 95)

Common errors in healthcare records include:

- records being illegible;
- records not being in chronological order;
- records not being contemporaneous;
- records not being signed by the person who made the entry;
- the date and timing of an entry not being recorded;
- records containing abbreviations, jargon or meaningless phrases;
- records not being made with the involvement of the patient or carer;
- patient or carer not being able to understand the content of the record;
- records not being factual, and containing speculation or subjective statements;
- the original entry having been altered, erased or deleted without a record of the change and information no longer being legible or visible;
- records not being stored in accordance with data protection legislation.

Further reading

Aggleton, P and Chalmers, H (2000) *Nursing Models and Nursing Practice*, 2nd edition. Basingstoke: Palgrave Macmillan.

This book contains an overview of the main models of nursing.

Brown, SJ (2009) *Evidence-based Nursing: The research–practice connection.* Sudbury, MA: Jones and Bartlett.

An easy-to-read text designed for nursing students, which explores how to engage in evidence-based practice.

Brown, J and Libberton, P (eds) (2007) *Principles of Professional Studies in Nursing.* Basingstoke: Palgrave Macmillan.

A useful text, which explores beliefs and values of nursing, management of care issues and evidence-based practice and clinical effectiveness.

Gerrish, K and Lacey, A (2006) *The Research Process in Nursing,* 5th edition. Oxford: Blackwell.

A slightly more advanced text, which explores principles of the research process.

Holland, K, Jenkins, J, Solomon, J and Whittam, S (eds) (2008) *Applying the Roper-Logan-Tierney Model in Practice.* Edinburgh: Churchill Livingstone Elsevier.

This book explores the use of the Roper-Logan-Tierney Model through the use of case studies and exercises. The text does have an adult nursing focus, but is a useful foundation for all fields.

Mallik, M, Hall, C and Howard, D (2009) *Nursing Knowledge and Practice,* 3rd edition. London: Baillière Tindall.

An excellent foundation text, which provides in-depth knowledge to enable students to deliver care.

Useful websites

http://cochrane.co.uk The Cochrane Collaboration is an international and independent organisation that produces contemporary accurate information about the effects of healthcare. It produces and disseminates systematic reviews of healthcare interventions and promotes the search for evidence in the form of clinical trials and other studies of interventions.

www.library.nhs.uk The NHS Evidence Health Information Resources website provides access to comprehensive health resources.

www.nice.org.uk The National Institute for Health and Clinical Excellence (NICE), which provides national guidance on promoting good health and preventing and treating ill health.

www.nmc-uk.org Nursing and Midwifery Council website.

www.pdptoolkit.co.uk Click on 'Evidence Based Medicine'. The Centre for Evidence Based Medicine develops, teaches and promotes evidence-based healthcare and provides support and resources to doctors and healthcare professionals to help maintain the highest standards of medicine.

Chapter 5
Nursing as a global health activity

Valerie Gorton

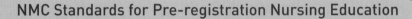

NMC Standards for Pre-registration Nursing Education

This chapter will address the following competences:

Domain 1: Professional values

3. All nurses must support and promote the health, wellbeing, rights and dignity of people, groups, communities and populations. These include people whose lives are affected by ill health, disability, ageing, death and dying. Nurses must understand how these activities influence public health.

4. All nurses must work in partnership with service users, carers, families, groups, communities and organisations. They must manage risk, and promote health and wellbeing while aiming to empower choices that promote self-care and safety.

5. All nurses must fully understand the nurse's various roles, responsibilities and functions, and adapt their practice to meet the changing needs of people, groups, communities and populations.

Domain 3: Nursing practice and decision making

3. All nurses must carry out comprehensive, systematic nursing assessments that take account of relevant physical, social, cultural, psychological, spiritual, genetic and environmental factors, in partnership with service users and others through interaction, observation and measurement.

4. All nurses must ascertain and respond to the physical, social and psychological needs of people, groups and communities. They must then plan, deliver and evaluate safe, competent, person-centred care in partnership with them, paying special attention to changing health needs during different life stages, including progressive illness and death, loss and bereavement.

5. All nurses must understand public health principles, priorities and practice in order to recognise and respond to the major causes and social determinants of health, illness and health inequalities. They must use a range of information and data to assess the needs of people, groups, communities and populations, and work to improve health, wellbeing and experiences of healthcare; secure equal access to health screening, health promotion and healthcare; and promote social inclusion.

> **Chapter aims**
>
> After reading this chapter, you should be able to:
>
> - understand the terms 'global nursing' and 'globalisation';
> - explain healthcare and nursing within the context of the EU and internationally;
> - understand the meaning of culture and the effects of this on individual and community healthcare;
> - seek out opportunities for elective experiences of learning outside the UK later in the course;
> - develop responsibility for your own learning.
>
> Note: Throughout this chapter, the term 'nursing' is used collectively, although this does embrace all four field specialities of nursing and midwifery.

Introduction

This chapter will help you to develop your knowledge of the global aspect of nursing and the opportunities available to develop and enhance your cultural knowledge and experiences. Nursing and healthcare in the twenty-first century must embrace the global concept of health and the effects of globalisation on worldwide health. You will be introduced to material that will assist you to explore your knowledge, values and beliefs in relation to global health issues.

It is intended that this chapter will encourage you to embrace the concepts of lifelong learning, career development and professional responsibility for your own learning. It will also introduce you to the opportunities for personal and professional development associated with elective experiences and learning outside the UK.

In October 2010, the UK Nursing and Midwifery Council introduced new standards for Nurse education allowing students to undertake academic or practice learning outside the UK for periods up to 6 months in duration. This is a radical change and it is proposed at this time that this will also apply to Midwifery education when the new Midwifery Standards for education are introduced in 2012. Some universities and approved education institutes (AEIs) may also offer short experience placements outside the home AEI but elsewhere within the UK. These changes allow more flexibility for education providers to include these opportunities within their programmes and this chapter aims to assist you in preparing for these.

Nursing as a global activity

The world is getting smaller – a mere five decades ago it used to take six weeks to reach Australia by boat and now it takes one day by air. This speed of travel makes the world readily accessible, resulting positively in an exchange of ideas, culture, skills and developments, and detrimentally in the rapid spread of diseases and the migration of healthcare workers, resulting in a concept called 'global health'. The World Health Organization (WHO), founded in 1948, is the authority on international health and first conceived the term 'global health'.

Each year WHO produces an annual report outlining key action points for that year. The 2007 report declared *A Safer Future: Global public health security in the 21st century* (WHO, 2007). One of WHO's key concerns in 2006 was the global movement of healthcare workers, which has in part increased the inequalities in health between countries as workers move from poorer to richer economies. The United Nations Millennium development goals are threatened in some poorer countries by the global shortage and mobility of healthcare workers. For the Western world, this international mobility should raise ethical and moral concerns, especially if the movement is not reciprocated in terms of professional skills, knowledge and education.

Perhaps focusing on the work and vision of WHO and others can assist us in grasping the concept of nursing as a global activity and the fact that no nation can act independently within the world as the actions of one country will impact on another.

> *Threats to health know no borders. In an age of widespread global trade and travel, new and existing diseases can cross national borders and threaten our collective security. Only through strong collaboration among developed and developing countries, together with an increased focus on information sharing and the strengthening of public health systems and surveillance, can we contain their spread.*
> (Chan, 2007)

Reflecting on this perspective, in 2008 the UK Government produced a five-year strategy entitled *Health is Global*. It is from this document that the definitions of 'global health' and 'globalisation' are taken for the content of this chapter.

Concept summary: Global health and globalisation

What is global health?

> *Global Health refers to health issues where the determinants circumvent, undermine or are oblivious to the territorial boundaries of states, and are thus beyond the capacity of individual countries to address through domestic institutions. Global health is focused on people across the whole planet rather than the concerns of particular nations. Global health recognises that health is determined by problems, issues and concerns that transcend national boundaries.*
> (DH, 2008a)

What is globalisation?

> *Globalisation is the widening or deepening and speeding up of worldwide interconnectedness in all aspects of contemporary social life. These global processes are changing the nature of human interaction across a wide range of social spheres including the economic, political, cultural and environmental.*
> (DH, 2008a)

Drawing from the consensus of opinion contained in these definitions, the developing world embraces the concept of globalisation defined by Scriven and Garman (2005) as *the increasing economic and social interdependence between countries* and the concept of global health as *recognis[ing] that health is determined by problems, issues and concerns that transcend national boundaries* (DH, 2008a).

The European Union (EU), to which the UK belongs, defines itself as:

a unique economic and political partnership between 27 democratic European countries whose aim is to bring peace, prosperity and freedom for its 495 million citizens – in a fairer, safer world.
(EU, 2008)

In the twenty-first century, nurses are educated for the global qualified healthcare professionals' resource. The changing demography of the global population is causing a widespread shortage of nurses. There is a definite shift from poorer, less developed countries to the richer countries of the Western world, which has a detrimental effect of diminishing qualified healthcare professionals in the poorer countries where they are most needed.

Activity 5.1   *Research and evidence-based practice*

To explore this a little further you can review the parliamentary debates highlighted in the links below.

Look at the discussions the politicians and professional bodies are having both in defining global health and also concerning the UK contribution to health and shared learning in developing countries.

Ask yourself who stands to gain or lose in these discussions.

*   Department of Health (DH, 2008a) *Health is Global: A UK Government strategy 2008–13* – **www.dh.gov.uk/en/Publicationsandstatistics/Publications/Publications PolicyAndGuidance/DH_088702**;
*   Department of Health (DH, 2007b) *Global Health Partnerships: The UK contribution to health in developing countries* – **www.dh.gov.uk/en/Publicationsandstatistics/ Publications/PublicationsPolicyAndGuidance/DH_065374**;
*   Department of Health (DH, 2004c) *Code of Practice for the International Recruitment of Healthcare Professionals* – **www.dh.gov.uk/en/Publicationsandstatistics/ Publications/PublicationsPolicyAndGuidance/DH_4097730**.
*   United Nations (2010) Summit on Millennium Development Goals – **http://www. un.org/milleniumgoals/**.

As this activity is based on your own research, there is no outline answer at the end of the chapter.

The effects of this on the profession of nursing are the comparability of nurse education within the EU and increased mobility of healthcare workers across the countries of the EU. Governments can contribute to global shortages of nurses by fair and equitable policies for migration and recruitment of qualified healthcare professionals. Opportunities for students to undertake studies in another country can only aid the reciprocity of this mobility and the understanding of health needs, conditions and structures in other countries.

Activity 5.2   *Reflection*

Reflecting on course content to date, identify any references to global health and global-isation.

Develop your own understanding of these terms.

As this activity is based on your own reflection, there is no outline answer at the end of the chapter.

Nurse education and the concept of global health

Nurse education is not only about achieving academic goals, but also about achieving professional and practice competencies, skills and knowledge to become a reflective, competent practitioner. At the beginning of training a student's first goal is to qualify and long-term career aspirations are usually formulated at a later stage in the education process. Professional and life experiences influence personal and professional career directions. The challenge is to recognise opportunities and to make the most of those opportunities. An essential skill, therefore, is to learn to take responsibility for your own learning and development. Within the concept of global health, it is essential that nursing knowledge is both learnt and applied within the context of cultural diversity and awareness.

The challenge for both students and nurse educators is how to facilitate the development of global nursing skills and competency acquisition, while still ensuring both academic credit accumulation and the quality of education.

Defining culture

It is from our own understanding of concepts that we are able to identify the knowledge needed to work with and within concepts as we pursue our nursing careers.

Culture related to global health activity

Often an education programme claims to address international issues through the subject of culture and it is culture within this context that we will now explore.

The term 'culture' has many diverse meanings. It can relate to:

- the aesthetic aspects of life, such as art, literature and music;
- an individual's values, beliefs and societal practices;
- society's morality, beliefs, social norms and behaviour;
- an individual's perception and understanding of his or her own world.

Reflecting on these diverse meanings, it is evident that culture can be studied and understood within either a narrow or broad dimension – a domestic or global context.

Culture within a domestic context can relate to learnt behaviour through personal experience within a family or society in which one lives or is reared.

Culture within a global context can embrace a whole range of different cultures, relating to other societies, countries or populations with all their inherent values and beliefs.

Activity 5.3   *Reflection*

Reflecting on course content to date, identify any references to culture and whether these have had a narrow or broad dimension.

Develop your own definition of culture in relation to your nursing practice and understanding of these terms.

As this activity is based on your own reflection, there is no outline answer at the end of the chapter.

Transcultural nursing

Transcultural nursing has been considered in relation to patient care for over four decades and was first articulated as a field of enquiry important to the culture of nursing by Leininger in the early 1950s (Ryan and Twibell, 2002). It is especially strong in the USA, where the population is more culturally diverse than here in the UK. However, the UK of the twenty-first century is a multicultural population and to ignore this subject within the field of nurse education programmes today is to ignore the different needs of cultural populations who are not indigenous to the UK.

Concept summary: What is transcultural nursing?

Within the practice of nursing and healthcare the term transcultural nursing implies:

> *a meeting of two or more cultures – the culture of the nursing profession, the nurse's own cultural background and the cultural background of the patient.*
> (Kenworthy et al., 2002, pp130–1)

Kenworthy's definition may be further expanded to include a fourth dimension, which is the culture of the environment within which care is delivered.

Andrews and Boyle (1995) suggest that transcultural care is an amalgam of different nursing and care concepts with some elements that are common across all cultures:

- *caring exists in all cultures;*
- *the way in which caring is carried out is culture specific;*
- *the meaning of caring varies cross-culturally;*
- *what constitutes care varies cross-culturally;*
- *where care matches client expectations, the more accepted it will be.*

(Cited in Kenworthy et al., 2002, p133)

Transcultural care focuses on worldwide cultures and the comparative effects of that cultural diversity on the cultures of caring, health and nursing (Papadopoulos, 2006). Papadopoulos believes that transcultural care is fundamental to the profession of nursing to develop 'culturally competent practitioners'. Nursing now embraces all cultures within both the workforce and the patient population, and healthcare should embrace a wide diversity of values and beliefs applied to the care a patient receives. Nurses trained within the UK are no longer only trained for the domestic market. As discussed earlier in this chapter, the mobility of healthcare workers inter-nationally is continuing to increase.

Challenges within the UK are to ensure that worldwide cultures and cultural diversity are paramount in all aspects of nursing education and care. The bio-medical model in nurse education lost its importance in the 1970s as a mechanistic model based on treatment of disease, and was replaced by a plethora of nursing models. However, in the most popularly applied models of nursing – Activities of Living (Roper et al., 1990; Henderson, 1966), Adaptation Model (Roy, 1970) and the Self-care Deficit Theory (Orem, 1985) – the cultural aspect of care as defined above is assumed and not clearly defined as a separate entity.

According to Kenworthy et al. (2002), cultural issues within nursing models are identified as being influencing factors on care under the *umbrella concept* of sociocultural factors, alongside other influencing factors, such as:

- biological factors;
- psychological factors;
- environmental factors;
- politico-economic factors.

The NMC clearly defines within its *Standards of Proficiency for Pre-registration Nursing Education* (NMC, 2004a) that all nurses must *provide a rationale for the nursing care delivered which takes account of social, cultural, spiritual, legal, political and economic influences.*

This is an all-embracing outcome, which states that cultural influences must underpin any nursing intervention. Duffy (2001) proposes that nurses have a moral obligation to provide care that includes culturally appropriate care.

From this discussion, it becomes clear that all student nurses must have a clear working definition of culture that will underpin future practice.

Activity 5.4   *Critical thinking*

Read around the subject of culture and re-examine the definition of culture that you previously identified.

Revise this definition in the light of your increased knowledge.

As this activity is based on your own reflection, there is no outline answer at the end of the chapter.

The integration of an elective experience, or learning outside the UK, within nursing programmes offers the student a real-life experience of another culture and its associated healthcare. It enables students to observe and understand the differing perceptions of health and disease within different cultures and social groups. Cultural awareness is best achieved through immersion in another culture, which can be achieved either in the UK or by working within another country. The rapidly increasing uses of information technology (IT) within nurse education programmes offers students opportunities for virtual reality experiences, but nothing can facilitate the exploration of feelings, values, beliefs and ethical issues like the total immersion within another culture and/or country.

Case study

Julia is a 28-year-old mother of four children under the age of ten years.

She is married to a subsistence farmer within the rural community of Tanzania. Her four children are survivors from her ten pregnancies and she has nursed, lost and grieved for six children during her short life.

The role of mother and wife is culturally defined and differs from that in the UK. Good health is defined as day-to-day survival, with all members of the family having enough to eat and drink.

Clean water in this environment is a goal of WHO, while malnutrition, gastro-intestinal infection, HIV/AIDS and death are constant enemies within Julia's life.

The WHO (1946) definition of health – *Health is a state of complete physical, mental and social well-being and not merely the absence of disease or infirmity* – was implemented worldwide in 1948 and has not changed since.

This definition is, therefore, all-embracing, but is seen by some as outdated for the twenty-first century. It does, however, set a standard for defining health on a global basis, especially in relation to the state of complete well-being.

Activity 5.5   *Reflection*

Reflect on Julia's case study and this extract from the DH report, *Global Health Partnerships*:

> *The contrasts with the UK are stark . . . Child deaths under five: in Sub-Saharan Africa, 179 in 1000; in UK 6 in 1,000 . . . Life expectancy for women in Sub-Saharan Africa 46, in UK 78 . . . Annual health expenditure per person: in Sub-Saharan Africa $36; in UK $2,508.*
> (DH, 2007b)

- What does the WHO definition of health mean to you?
- Is it still relevant in the twenty-first century?

As this activity is based on your own reflection, there is no outline answer at the end of the chapter.

However, 60 years later there are still vast inequalities in health across the world. In the UK in 1980, the Black Report concluded that there were still *persistent internal inequalities of health* (DHSS, 1980) in spite of 35 years of the NHS.

Likewise, WHO in its 2008 annual report concluded:

> *For fair and efficient systems, all people must have access to health care according to need and regardless of ability to pay. If they do not have access, health inequities produce decades of differences in life expectancies not only between countries but within countries. These inequities raise risks, especially of disease outbreaks, for all.*
> (WHO, 2008)

The WHO now states on its introductory web page that *In the 21st century, health is a shared responsibility, involving equitable access to essential care and collective defence against transnational threats* (WHO, 2011).

Activity 5.6   *Research and evidence-based practice*

To explore this a little further you can review the previously visited parliamentary debates and the WHO website highlighted in the links below.

- Department of Health (DH, 2008a) *Health is Global: A UK Government strategy 2008–13* – **www.dh.gov.uk/en/Publicationsandstatistics/Publications/Publications PolicyAndGuidance/DH_088702**;
- Department of Health (DH, 2007b) *Global Health Partnerships: The UK contribution to health in developing countries* – **www.dh.gov.uk/en/Publicationsandstatistics/ Publications/PublicationsPolicyAndGuidance/DH_065374**;
- World Health Organisation – **www.who.int**.

As this activity is based on your own observations, there is no outline answer at the end of the chapter.

It is, therefore, the responsibility of all nurse educators and all students of nursing to be cognisant of the differences in health equality, and develop knowledge and skills to minimise these within their scope of professional practice.

Student learning

Nurse education programmes within the UK are competency driven (**www.nmc-uk.org**). This means that, although every approved education institution (AEI) can determine an individual structure, within the 3-year degree programme, the competences achieved at the end must be common across all courses and are in fact the criteria for entry to the NMC professional register. Many AEIs will meet the needs for students to understand the needs of patients from other cultures within the population demography of their own NHS Trusts. However, this does not enable the students to experience an alternative culture of healthcare for themselves, or to experience cultures outside their own geographic area. In the current climate of the NHS, when students may not always seek or find employment within their own country, the time is right to educate nurses for travelling or seeking employment internationally.

Throughout your nurse preparation programme you will embark on a journey of learning. Through this journey you will learn to enquire, understand, reflect and identify learning deficits. This learning journey is not time limited to the duration of your formal education programme, but continues throughout your career through the concept of lifelong learning. The degree to which you embrace global health and globalisation will depend in part on your curriculum content, your experiences and your desire to learn.

In the usual scheme of things, a clinical practice is selected, organised and arranged by the learning experience office within the university in which the course is located. Applying to undertake an elective experience means that you are in control of your own learning. You can select the type of experience you would like and where you would like it to be, and define your own reasons for choosing this experience and the learning outcomes that you intend to achieve through this experience.

While the reasons for this must be clearly educationally defined and determined, this activity will assist you in developing the skills of lifelong learning and responsibility for your own learning.

Activity 5.7   *Reflection*

Consider that you would like to undertake an elective experience.

Spend some time writing a rationale and defining your own learning outcomes for this experience.

Where might you like to go? Why? What will you learn?

Outline answers are given at the end of the chapter.

An elective experience, either overseas or outside your university or home AEI, is a challenging and rewarding experience. It is not, however, always an essential integral component of pre-registration nurse education programmes. There will be some universities that do not participate in this activity and some which include this for all students.

Internationalising the curriculum

AEIs have responded to the need to internationalise their curricula through a variety of methods. Among these participating AEIs, each will offer slightly different experiences or opportunities. These can take the form of:

- full semester exchange, both academic or practice learning;
- short period exchange, practice learning.

The ERASMUS Scheme (European Community Action Scheme for the Mobility of University Students) is one of the European Commission's educational schemes for students, teachers and institutions. It was introduced in 1987 with the aim of increasing student mobility within the European Union (EU, 1987). The EU consisted of 12 member states in 1987 and in 2007 there were 27 members states, with several more countries identified as ascension countries for entry in 2008 (EU, 2008). As ERASMUS celebrated its twentieth anniversary in 2007, a total of 31 countries in Europe participated in the ERASMUS course and now 150,000 people benefit from ERASMUS exchanges every year (EC, 2007).

Why undertake an elective learning experience?

ERASMUS benefits (results from ERASMUS research)

Top 10 reasons to take part in an ERASMUS programme are:

- to stand out in the job market – a great addition to your CV;
- to return more motivated, independent and confident;
- to get a grant;
- it counts towards your course; it is not a gap year;
- to learn a range of life skills not taught in the lecture theatre;
- to access a wider range of subject areas than in the UK;
- to improve your language skills;
- to gain an international network of friends and meet your lifelong partner;
- to discover a different culture and gain an international perspective;
- it's really good fun.

(**www.britishcouncil.org/erasmus**)

This offers opportunities for nursing students to participate in ERASMUS exchanges within Europe and brings with it support for students to assist with financing this opportunity. However, there are constraints to this scheme that will be explored later in this chapter.

The Bologna Process (EC, 1999) called for *harmonisation of educational qualification systems in Europe.* Six action points were identified to achieve this. These are:

* adoption of a system of easily readable and comparable degrees;
* a system of two-cycle degrees;
* a system of credits to promote widespread student mobility;
* promotion of student mobility;
* promotion of European cooperation in quality assurance;
* promotion of the European dimension in higher education.

In 2001, the Prague Declaration added three more action points, which are:

* emphasis on lifelong learning;
* involvement of students in AEIs;
* enhancement of the attractiveness and competitiveness of A higher education in Europe to other parts of the world.

In 2000, the Lisbon Agenda stated that the EU should become *the most dynamic and competitive knowledge-based economy in the world capable of sustainable economic growth with more and better jobs and greater social cohesion, and respect for the environment by 2010,* thus encouraging mobility of the workforce throughout the EU.

EU member states have continued to meet on a biannual basis at summit meetings under the title of the Bologna Process and have since set a target date of 2010 for these nine action points and the Lisbon Agenda to be achieved. In line with the expansion of worldwide enhancement of the EU, representatives of Australia, New Zealand and the USA have attended these later summit meetings and are examining the adoption of the Bologna Process aims into their own country's education systems.

Referring back to the concept of nursing as a global health activity, it would appear that cross-cultural, cross-country experiences should be fully embraced by student nurses during their education programmes. There are clear benefits to students undertaking this experience.

Activity 5.8   *Decision making*

Imagine you were planning to undertake an elective experience; write down a rationale and five learning outcomes that would contribute to your own professional and personal development.

As this activity is based on your own reflection and observation, there is no outline answer at the end of the chapter.

Benefits of elective experiences

Elective experiences enable individuals not only to learn within a changing environment and culture, but also to apply previously learnt knowledge and acquired skills to influence change within a new environment.

Some students may see this as a pleasure-seeking opportunity and not a pure learning opportunity or objective; however, a truly self-directed learner will perceive the opportunities for learning outweighing the opportunities for having fun. This does not mean that learning and fun are incompatible, but that learning should be fun, which in turn increases motivation levels and the level of learning (Gorton, 2004).

Cultural awareness

Cultural awareness is best achieved through immersion in another culture. An elective experience can be undertaken either overseas, or within the UK, within a more culturally diverse population. The UK is becoming an increasingly multicultural society and across the UK the diversity of the population varies considerably (**www.statistics.gov.uk**). Students who cannot afford an overseas elective would benefit from experiencing care in a different cultural environment, especially if your 'home' Trust is located in a rural or predominantly indigenous population area.

Travel

'Travel broadens the mind' is a commonly held belief and underpins the concept of the student 'gap year'. Unfortunately, many nursing students do not have the opportunity to undertake a gap year prior to commencing nurse education and electives give students the opportunity to rectify this in part. The concept of travel as a part of the educational growing-up process has been fully embraced by the USA, Canada and Australia for many years, and students who do not travel are in the minority, which is contrary to the UK, where students who travel are in the minority.

Increased student motivation

Identification of your own learning needs and participation in the what, when, how and where learning takes place raises your levels of motivation to learn.

- Adults want to be successful learners.
- Adults want to feel a choice in their learning.
- Adults want to learn something they value.
- Adults want to experience the learning as pleasurable.

Responsibility for own learning

Being prepared to take responsibility for yourself and your learning is the key to lifelong learning. Qualified nurses are required by the NMC to demonstrate lifelong learning each time they re-register to practise (NMC, 2004a). This evidence is presented in a professional portfolio, which demonstrates learning experiences, reflections and plans for future action. Many nurse education programmes included professional portfolio development as an integral part of the nurse education course and assessment process. An elective experience offers students a choice of geographical location and an opportunity to define their own learning outcomes to meet their individual needs, sometimes in addition to course-set objectives. This learning experience can be evidenced in the professional portfolio and can then be utilised in career development and selection interviews to demonstrate a wider interest and knowledge base, and application of learning to an alternative environment.

Case study

Nursing models formulate the structure for history, taking in all nursing interventions. Roper et al.'s Activities of Living Model (1983; 2000) offers a tried and tested model used widely in the UK.

An elective experience in Malta demonstrated to students that the medical model of care was still paramount. Reflecting on this model, students identified problems for nurses, focusing on their professional autonomy and development.

Reflecting on this scenario, were patients in Malta in danger of deprivation of nursing expertise that falls outside the medical model of care?

Personal development

Nursing students develop both personally and professionally during their education programmes and their clinical experiences. Their own individual values and beliefs are questioned through the clinical experiences. However, the education process alone does not always offer life-changing experiences. Travelling with a group on a package holiday to a popular destination cannot equate to travelling alone or with a colleague to work in another culture or country. Each time you change a clinical experience within your 'home' experience circuit, you are challenged with new environments, new relationships and a new working culture. The challenges of an elective are all these and more. Experience has demonstrated that students who undertake electives are confident and have well-developed decision-making and application skills.

Widening horizons

Student nurses do not always travel to a new location to undertake their education programmes, nor do they live away from home. The percentage of nurses who train near their home towns is higher than in other university courses. The geographical location of your practice can influence your future career and your knowledge base and skills, even though the outcome of your course will be a knowledgeable, competent nurse practitioner. Elective experiences offer the opportunity to work in an alternative environment – country, town, urban location, rural location, diverse population, etc. Any of these will offer a wider experience and diversity of opportunities. An elective can also be seen as an opportunity to explore an alternative employment opportunity, for example, a trial experience in Australia prior to emigrating, or a trial experience with the armed forces prior to applying to enlist.

Challenges, concerns and constraints of elective experiences

Obversely, there are some challenges, concerns and constraints for every student being able to take advantage of these opportunities.

Language

Populations who speak English as their first language are often reluctant to try acquiring other languages, which is certainly apparent within the UK.

- UK school curricula have not historically prioritised language acquisition in the choice of subjects offered, though this is beginning to change.
- Nurse preparation programmes do not normally have enough flexibility to enable language acquisition to be an optional part of the programme, even though most universities have language units, skills and resources to facilitate this development.

Mature student population

The UK has encouraged mature applicants into nurse education programmes, valuing their life skills and commitment, which can bring different challenges, such as:

- responsibilities for children and/or dependants;
- less disposable income.

Financial implications

Nursing students undertaking a diploma education course will be receiving a bursary payment, which will continue while they undertake an elective experience. Nursing students undertaking a degree course will not receive a bursary and are on student loans or grants. Increasingly, nurse education programmes are being taught at degree level in line with EU aspirations. Either way, no student receives a large amount of money during their programme.

- This results in a shortfall for travel and self-funded opportunities.
- ERASMUS offers students a lump sum to assist with these costs if the exchange opportunity is for a period of 12 weeks or more and lies within the EU with an ERASMUS partner institution.
- Course commitments often make working extra hours to earn extra funds demanding.

Fear of the unknown

Travelling to another country as a leisure activity is exciting, but engaging in work in an alternative culture and country is challenging, demanding and stressful.

- Recently acquired nursing skills are tested and applied to new situations.
- Procedures, protocols and legislation are different.

- Familiarity and the security of family, friends and tutors are far away.
- Email and telephone communications do not fully compensate for loss of face-to-face interaction.

Student elective experiences

Reciprocal exchanges set the whole exchange process within a legislative framework, clearly identifying roles and responsibilities for hosts in both countries.

The NMC (2010) has enabled universities and AEIs to structure nurse education programmes more flexibly to include short periods of no longer than four weeks elective experience, which will be formatively assessed, and a longer period of academic and practice learning of up to six months outside the UK, which will be summatively assessed. However, this still offers HEIs some challenges in matching course content, structure and timing across partners:

- different AEI semester and course dates in different countries;
- different academic content;
- ensuring the quality of mentor supervision in practical settings;
- ensuring reciprocal quality assurance mechanisms for award of credits;
- mismatch between learning outcomes.

None of these are insurmountable but do require 'thinking outside the box' to overcome. The key word to making these experiences work is 'flexibilty' not only on the part of the educational institution, but also of the student. Students need to be flexible, willing to move an annual leave week to accommodate an elective experience.

Achievement of learning outcomes should be achievable in a variety of settings.

Culture shock

Adjusting to your new surroundings may take time . . . :

> *Studying and living in a new country is an exciting and rewarding experience. Nevertheless, there may be times that you feel anxious or homesick because there are many things around you that are unfamiliar. Do not worry – it is quite usual to experience some sort of 'culture shock'. Make sure you keep in touch with friends and family at home, but also find out about and join in the social life at your new university. There will be many people around you who will be able to offer you explanations, friendship and support.*
> (Lowes, et al., 2004, pp301–2)

However, one of the learning outcomes of the whole elective experience is to embrace another culture. The extent to which you experience culture shock will be determined by the breadth of differences between your own comfort zone, normal cultural experiences, and the new culture you are embracing.

Activity 5.9   *Reflection*

Imagine you are considering an elective experience.

- What preparation would you need?
- What questions would you want to ask?

Outline answers are given at the end of the chapter.

'Where there's a will, there's a way' – if we have the determination to do something, we can always find the path or method to do it – an old proverb that is worth remembering by both students and academics.

Not all students, though, will be able to embrace the opportunity of elective experience in another country due to some of the constraints indicated above.

Alternative opportunities may still present themselves to these students. These include:

- combining holiday experience with work experience;
- taking an elective within the UK within a more culturally diverse setting.

Combining holiday experience with work experience

A large percentage of students, whether studying nursing or other disciplines, will take a package holiday overseas during the course of their training. This can either be sun-soaked beach relaxation or an opportunity to experience the culture of another country. There are opportunities to combine the two so that you absorb some of the cultural experiences and apply these to healthcare and nursing in the future.

Think of the environmental issues and the influences on health – housing, water, education, health services. As a tourist one is often sheltered from these influences, but a little exploration can lead to a lot of information.

Alternatively, there are opportunities for students to undertake a working experience abroad with organisations such as BUNAC or Real Gap Experience.

Summer Camp USA offers eligible applicants a chance for a fun and worthwhile summer living alongside and working with children aged 6–16 on summer camp in the USA or Canada.
(**www.bunac.org**)

Community Development Work India
By joining a community development project in a village in India you will have a great cultural experience which is authentic and rewarding. The work will be fun and challenging, and you will be experiencing true Indian culture whilst assisting in bringing attention to the facilities and social issues of the village.
(**www.realgap.co.uk**)

Or search the web for other ideas for a few weeks' or months' experience. It may not be possible to do what you want to do during your course, but it may be at the end. Some experiences are paid and some are voluntary.

Take an elective within the UK in a more culturally diverse setting

The UK is not only a multicultural society, but is now considered to be a multifaith society. Both these elements – culture and faith – can influence healthcare from the perspectives of prevention, health promotion, diagnosis, treatment and aftercare. A nurse preparation programme undertaken in a rural area with a mainly indigenous population offers the student different experiences from a nurse preparation programme undertaken in the centre of a large city. All students will achieve the competences required by the NMC, but the application of these competences and the experience gained will vary. Students who cannot afford an overseas elective would benefit from experiencing care in a different cultural environment. The challenge is sometimes to find an alternative that is both accessible and offers you the alternative learning experience that you require. The UK Government website (**www.statistics.gov.uk**) will outline the breakdown of the population in any given area, and accessing the websites for the health services in a particular geographical area will give an insight into the services offered and the health issues that predominate in that area.

Assessment of elective experiences

Assessment of elective experiences varies with each AEI and the different agreements that are formulated between them and their elective partners. However, the mentorship of all nurse education students is clearly defined for a first-level nurse in every practice setting. The assessment of an elective can also be further complicated by the transfer of credits achieved in another organisation and each AEI has different rules and regulations relating to this. Students should be aware of the processes for their own AEI.

> *The primary aim in pre-registration nursing programmes is to ensure that students are prepared to practise safely and effectively to such an extent that the protection of the public is assured.*
> (**www.nmc-uk.org**)

To this end, most elective experiences take place during the third year of the course when a large range of basic clinical skills has been acquired.

Developing a professional portfolio to evidence elective experience

A portfolio is a live and dynamic document, designed specifically for extracting and inserting relevant clinical and theoretical information to evidence your achievement. It is an opportunity for you to integrate theory and practice in a way that is most relevant to you as an individual. A portfolio can be used as a whole document to evidence your progression throughout the whole three years of your course, or used to evidence individual separate pieces or stages of your development. In this instance, it will be used to evidence the achievement of your learning outcomes during an elective experience.

During an elective you will be bombarded with new experiences and feelings every day. Therefore, it is a good idea to keep the following in mind.

- The construction of a portfolio can seem daunting, but it need not be. You need to remember that there is no right or wrong way to construct a portfolio, provided that you can justify the structure that you have chosen. The evidence within your portfolio demonstrates your learning from theory and its application to practice (Reed, 2011). This is never more important than in the elective experience, where you are applying previously learnt knowledge to new cultures and environments.

- A journal or diary is a good way to keep track of events and affords some structure to your reflections and subsequent learning. Although the structure of your portfolio to evidence learning outcomes may be in the form of the NMC domains, a diary or journal can assist you to encompass those valuable feelings and experiences that do not clearly fit into a domain or learning outcome, but that, when measured together, contribute to the overall learning experience that has demonstrated your personal and professional development.

- Personal reflections on any learning experience are a good aide-memoire for you when you come to compile your final professional portfolio. It is worth remembering that experiences that may not be measured or assessed at this stage of the course can be useful for future assessments and/or future employment interviews or opportunities.

Student feedback

It was awesome; I am so overwhelmed; Thank you so much for arranging this experience for me.
(four-week experience, USA)

Thank you for this fantastic opportunity to visit and work in such a fantastic country. The experience has been amazing and will stay with me for the rest of my life.
(eight-week experience, Australia)

Overall the experience was a massive positive experience and I would encourage any other student thinking about going to do it to stop thinking and do it.
(six-week experience, Australia)

Everyone has made us so welcome and I have learnt so much.
(six-week experience, Sweden)

I thoroughly enjoyed my experience and found the experience extremely useful to my future practice as I have found most of the skills I learnt will be transferable to my NHS practice.
(four-week experience, UK)

Overall a fantastic learning experience. Every member of staff was proactive in my learning.
(four-week experience, UK)

This experience has enhanced my knowledge whilst working alongside nurses on the ward, clinic and in community. I have developed my knowledge of different aspects of nursing care which will be of enormous benefit for my future practice as a nurse.
(four-week experience, UK)

Conclusion

In a classic definition, Burton (1963) identifies learning as:

> *A change in the individual, due to the interaction between that individual, and his environment, which fills*
> *a need and makes him more capable of dealing adequately with his environment.*
> (Cited in Knowles et al., 1998, p12)

The journey through this chapter will hopefully have filled a need in your knowledge and will inspire you to consider the global implications of healthcare and the opportunities available to you not only to experience healthcare in alternative cultures and countries, but also to influence your future healthcare practice.

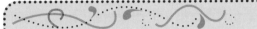

Chapter summary

This chapter has enabled you to develop your knowledge of the global aspect of nursing and the opportunities available to develop and enhance your cultural knowledge and experiences. You have been introduced to material that will assist you to explore your knowledge, values and beliefs in relation to global health issues.

It was intended that this chapter would encourage you to embrace the concepts of lifelong learning, career development and professional responsibility for your own learning. The concept of elective experiences, to expand your personal and professional development, has been explored in relation to the benefits, concerns, challenges and constraints of such experiences. As you progress in your nursing career, this knowledge will enable you to identify shortfalls in your cultural knowledge and pursue opportunities for elective experience to equip you for nursing in the twenty-first century, both within the UK and internationally.

Activities: brief outline answers

Activity 5.7 (page 107)

Sample rationale
An elective learning experience in . . . will expand my clinical skills and knowledge, as this is an area of nursing that I wish to work in post-qualifying. I have a particular interest in understanding the social and cultural influences on healthcare. Previously learnt knowledge and skills will be applied in a different healthcare setting and I feel this will offer me a valuable experience.

Where might you like to go?
- Seriously consider this point. Do not pick a country or experience that would appear to give you an experience that no one else has had, but one that will contribute to your overall nursing skills and knowledge.

Why?
- Clearly define your learning outcomes.
- Make sure the statements can be evidenced in your professional portfolio.

What will you learn?

- Identify clinical skills and knowledge, and those extra elements that you have identified in your rationale.

Activity 5.9 (page 114)

What preparation would you need?

- Research the country or area of the UK that you would like to undertake your elective in.
- Clearly identify the reasons why you want to undertake an elective in that place.
- Write a rationale and your learning outcomes to focus your thoughts.

What questions would you want to ask?

- How much will it cost?
- Can I afford it?
- Where will I live?
- Do I want to travel alone?
- Will I miss home?
- Do I get on with the person I am going with?

- Will the experience meet my learning outcomes and benefit my future career development?
- Will it be safe?
- Will it affect my assessment of theory or practice and my course progression?

Further reading

Kenworthy, N, Snowley, G and Gilling, C (2002) *Common Foundation Studies in Nursing*. Edinburgh: Churchill Livingstone.

Good, basic introductory textbook.

Pearson, A, Vaughan, B and Fitzgerald, M (2004) *Nursing Models for Practice*. London: Macmillan.

A clear and accessible guide to different theories and models of nursing.

Reed, S (2011) *Successful Professional Porfolios for Nursing Students*. Exeter: Learning Matters.

Everything you need to know about how and why to put a professional portfolio together.

Useful websites

www.bunac.org BUNAC arranges international gap year and holiday opportunities for university students.

www.erasmus.ac.uk Website of ERASMUS, the lifelong learning scheme for HE students, outlining funding opportunities.

http://europa.eu/abc/panorama/index_en.htm An introduction to the EU, together with its current policies and procedures.

www.nmc-uk.org The website of the NMC, on which you can find the competencies for nursing education.

www.realgap.co.uk Real Gap organises gap year experiences for students.

www.statistics.gov.uk Census results and collated statistics for the UK.

www.who.int Official website of the World Health Organization; includes mission statements, project work, policies, etc.

Chapter 6
Being qualified

Gill Langmack

NMC Standards for Pre-registration Nursing Education

This chapter will address the following competencies:

Domain 1: Professional values

1. All nurses must practise with confidence according to *The Code: Standards of conduct, performance and ethics for nurses and midwives* (NMC 2008a), and within other recognised ethical and legal frameworks. They must be able to recognise and address ethical challenges relating to people's choices and decision making about their care, and act within the law to help them and their families and carers find acceptable solutions.

2. All nurses must practise in a holistic, non-judgmental, caring and sensitive manner that avoids assumptions, supports social inclusion; recognises and respects individual choice; and acknowledges diversity. Where necessary, they must challenge inequality, discrimination and exclusion from access to care.

Domain 3: Nursing practice and decision making

1. All nurses must use up-to-date knowledge and evidence to assess, plan, deliver and evaluate care, communicate findings, influence change and promote health and best practice. They must make person-centred, evidence-based judgments and decisions, in partnership with others involved in the care process, to ensure high quality care. They must be able to recognise when the complexity of clinical decisions requires specialist knowledge and expertise, and consult or refer accordingly.

Domain 4: Leadership, management and team working

Generic Standard: All nurses must be professionally accountable and use clinical governance processes to maintain and improve nursing practice and standards of healthcare. They must be able to respond autonomously and confidently to planned and uncertain situations, managing themselves and others effectively. They must create and maximise opportunities to improve services. They must also demonstrate the potential to develop further management and leadership skills during their period of preceptorship and beyond.

Chapter aims

After reading this chapter, you will be able to:

- define the key changes in qualifying as a first-level nurse;
- discuss the major concerns of many newly qualified nurses;
- determine the major support mechanisms available post qualification;
- identify the practicalities of finding and getting your first nursing post;
- identify the main practicalities to consider in being employed as a nurse;
- understand your own role and challenges in qualifying.

Introduction

This chapter looks specifically at what it's like to qualify as a nurse at the end of a nursing degree course. What are the worries and the concerns newly qualified nurses have and how can the various initiatives available help make the transition to a qualified, skilled and practising nurse a smooth one? As earlier chapters have explored, nursing involves a multitude of different skills requiring extensive knowledge and understanding to care for and manage often very different and potentially challenging situations. Nursing models and frameworks are used to assess clients, prioritise, plan and evaluate nursing care, while other tools aid reflection on situations. Providing good nursing care depends on learning clinical skills, delivering those skills safely, appropriately and effectively, and supporting the patient or client on an individual basis. At the point of qualifying, there are additional issues to consider.

Activity 6.1   *Reflection*

Think about a skill you have learnt during your earlier years – something that took you some time to learn, for example learning to swim, learning to drive a car, becoming good at numeracy at school – learning your times tables perhaps.

- Think back to when you were learning the skill. How did it feel to be constantly trying, yet knowing that you hadn't fully mastered the skill?
- How did it feel at the point at which you could think – Yes, I've cracked it – I *can* do it?
- Once you felt confident to do the skill, how did it then feel to do it without help and support, maybe showing someone else who hadn't yet been able to achieve the same degree of success as you?

An outline answer is given at the end of the chapter.

What is it like to qualify?

Although all the tools of nursing can be explored in nurse education and, to continue with the 'vehicle' analogy of Chapters 3 and 4, the 'mechanic' can ensure the vehicle is working properly before you start it up, it relies on you, the nurse, or the driver, to drive the vehicle properly, following the rules of the road, putting your training into practice.

Finally achieving a much longed-for goal is immensely satisfying – feeling proud, both of yourself and of your colleagues who achieved their nurse registration at the same time. Yet, there is also a part that can feel scared – scared about 'messing it up'; scared about the unknown.

This doesn't mean that new nurses will know and have experienced absolutely everything there is to know about nursing patients and clients at the point at which they achieve their registration. It means that nurses are able to prioritise, plan, deliver and evaluate nursing care that is appropriate to their patients in a safe, timely and coordinated way, and are able to communicate effectively with all the agencies appropriate to the care of their patient or client. It also means they can show understanding of the rationale for the care they plan and give, as required by the patient or client. It means, too, that they have experienced a range of approaches they can use to plan nursing care, which can be tailored to the individual needs of specific patient(s). It doesn't mean, though, that they necessarily feel confident in using all those different approaches that they are aware of. Finally, it does mean that new nurses have developed and continue to develop professional attitudes to care, awareness of their responsibilities and an accountability in providing evidence-based care.

Activity 6.2   *Reflection*

Read through the following case study and reflect on how you might feel if you were put in this situation.

Case study

Jess is currently a third-year nurse on her management learning experience. She is about to complete the course in the next two weeks and has been feeling extremely apprehensive about the process. She knows she's passed all her assignments and she's going to get her degree – a 2:2, about which she's very proud, but there's a nagging doubt. She goes on to the general surgical ward each day and is given a group of patients to look after. She prioritises their care, discusses the issues with each individual patient and then supports those patients through the shift. She asks her mentor to help her with checking and giving medications and generally feels confident in undertaking the care required.

Jess took charge of this ward yesterday, though, and felt completely out of her depth. As the 'person in charge of the ward', Jess had to answer queries from the medical staff, and was an active member of the ward round – the ward was full with numerous admissions and discharges. Jess had a good complement of nurses on shift, so her mentor was able to

continued overleaf . . .

continued . . . •••

work closely with her. Halfway into the shift, Jess had one patient who returned from theatre following an operation and who bled unexpectedly post-operatively. Jess urgently needed to find medical support prior to her patient returning to theatre. The patient's wife was distraught at her husband needing to return to theatre. Thankfully, he returned about an hour later and had no further post-operative problems, but Jess went home from the shift feeling very relieved that the shift had finished and unsure about her own practical abilities, reflecting on the degree of help she had needed to sort the problems that had occurred.

Problems like these had been discussed to an extent in class and Jess had listened to the ensuing discussions, but being a part of the situation had meant she had to react to what was happening and, more than that, she'd needed to ring other departments to organise her patient's return to theatre – porters, theatres and medical staff. Jess's mentor had opted to talk to the gentleman's wife, for which Jess was extremely thankful. She couldn't think what to say to support her and help her to calm down. Once the problem was resolved, the busy ward still needed managing, so Jess was unable to sit and reflect on the whole situation until she finished the shift. Jess felt she'd been over-reliant on her mentor, who she felt had been fantastic, telling Jess who to ring next, reassuring her and generally being very supportive.

As Jess's mentor was unable to stay and reflect on the situation immediately following the shift, Jess and her mentor had agreed to meet up the following day at work and reflect more fully on the situation and responses that had been made.

An outline answer is given at the end of the chapter.

Jess's experience is not uncommon, as managing a group of patients or the ward and experiencing the practicalities in troubleshooting problems is a skill that only starts to be learnt on management placements. Remember that, for some students, opportunities to troubleshoot problems may not occur until after they qualify. It's not possible to experience the myriad of problems and issues that can occur.

Newly qualified nurses may be extremely nervous as they start their first post as a qualified nurse and feel that they've lost all the knowledge and skills learnt as a student. The feeling of now being responsible and accountable, with the expectation that the nurse will work independently, means that asking questions can feel like failing. Gaining confidence and experience over the first six months will help the newly registered nurse to feel more settled. Anecdotally, for some this is a natural progression and a straightforward extension of their role as a student, particularly for those who start working in an area where they also did their management experience (Clark and Holmes, 2007).

Research summary

This section identifies some of the current research, but you may wish to follow this up further – see the 'Further reading' section at the end of the chapter.

While there are some quantitative studies, in understanding the issues for the newly qualified nurse, it is more useful to identify common issues arising from relevant qualitative studies. These take either a phenomenological approach to understand what it is like to be newly qualified (Ramritu and Barnard, 2001; Jackson, 2005; O'Shea and Kelly, 2007; Hartigan et al., 2010) or an inductive, ground theory approach identifying the common themes that occur within a group of newly qualified nurses (Gerrish, 2000; Rungapadiachy et al., 2006; Mooney, 2007). Kramer (1974) identified a 'reality shock' for nurses in situations they had not experienced previously.

Themes arising from the research include:

* concerns about clinical skills (Gerrish, 2000; Clark and Holmes, 2007; O'Shea and Kelly, 2007; Hartigan et al., 2010);
* developing confidence (Clark and Holmes, 2007; O'Shea and Kelly, 2007);
* feeling supported (Gerrish, 2000; O'Shea and Kelly, 2007);
* making care and treatment errors (Ramritu and Barnard, 2001; Ross and Clifford, 2002); individual accountability (Gerrish, 2000; Clark and Holmes, 2007);
* adapting to the new role (Clark and Holmes, 2007; O'Shea and Kelly, 2007);
* less patient contact, so an increase in non-nursing duties (O'Shea and Kelly,2007);
* managerial responsibilities (Gerrish, 2000; O'Shea and Kelly, 2007);
* mentoring student nurses (O'Shea and Kelly, 2007).

Interestingly, interviewing nurses at around six months post-qualifying appears to be the point at which there has been enough time to settle into the role and to start to develop some confidence (Maben and Macleod Clark, 1998; Gerrish, 2000; Maben et al., 2006). However, authors have also identified this time as the point at which the sheer enormity of the role becomes apparent (Hole, 2005).

Research carried out with nurses who had been qualified around 10–12 months identifies yet more issues in addition to those seen above. These include:

* ethical considerations (Ramritu and Barnard, 2001);
* improved relationships with patients (Jackson, 2005);
* gaps between the nurse's knowledge and ability to practise (Khomeiran et al., 2006);
* possible ambiguity in the role (Gerrish, 2000; O'Connor et al., 2001; Rungapadiachy et al., 2006; Mooney, 2007).

Research studies clearly identify a need for clarity in what is expected by the newly qualified nurse in terms of having appropriate knowledge and skills. They also show that not all nurses feel fully prepared to practise autonomously at the point of registration (Ross and Clifford, 2002; Jackson, 2005; Maben et al., 2007; Mooney, 2007; Clark and Holmes, 2007;

Ball and Pike, 2007; Danbjørg and Birkelund, 2011). There are feelings of anxiety and a lack of confidence when starting their first nursing post – worries that are echoed at times by experienced, qualified staff (Maben et al., 2006; Lofmark et al., 2006; Clark and Holmes, 2007). What is evident, anecdotally, is that, in gaining confidence, the newly qualified nurse is able to pick and use the skills he or she has to ensure that the care given is excellent.

Achieving the requisite knowledge and clinical skills and, in particular, developing confidence takes time. For some students, three years' education is too much, while, for many others, it is far too short to take on all the information they feel they need to now.

There is a need to recognise limitations and to understand that becoming qualified is only the start of a professional career as a nurse. At the point at which the student completes their nurse education, and is able to register as a qualified nurse, they will have successfully achieved all their exams, assignments and shown a consistent ability to work effectively in different and varied learning experience areas. At this point the student nurse will have been assessed by the university where they are doing the course as being 'fit for practice', 'fit for purpose' and 'fit for the award' given.

Starting that first nursing job as a qualified nurse in an area where, as a student, the nurse did their final practice experience, may feel less of a difference than getting a job in a different area, such as in the community, or in different hospitals within this country or abroad (Clark and Holmes, 2007). This is likely to be due to the knowledge and skills they gained as a student through the final management experience in understanding the issues and practising the skills required by patients or clients.

The Department of Health (DH, 2006) identifies four elements of the nurse's role as:

1. practice issues/clinical skills;
2. leadership, management and supervision;
3. quality and service development;
4. education, training and development.

Activity 6.3 — *Reflection*

As you read through the following list based on the four elements identified above, think about how these elements apply to your own thoughts about working as a newly qualified nurse.

As this activity is based on your own reflection, there is no outline answer at the end of the chapter.

Practice issues/clinical skills

Nursing care is multifaceted and becomes more complex as the nurse grows in confidence and experience. The newly qualified nurse, therefore, should expect to need to assess the healthcare needs of patients, communicating and collaborating with the multiprofessional team and supporting the development of strategies to provide individualised care (Gerrish, 2000; Edmond, 2001). This will involve making reasoned judgements on the health and ability of patients or clients to help develop or maintain their independence based on sound knowledge, best evidence and local protocols.

Providing healthcare for some patients or clients requires complex decision making, for example in supporting and empowering patients requiring rehabilitation. As identified in Activity 6.2, there is a need to develop abilities to be able to 'read a situation' and to understand what is happening, much of which can only come through experience (Edmond, 2001).

Nurse education provides knowledge and skills training to undertake specific clinical skills, for example in changing a person's dressing on a wound using a non-touch, aseptic technique. While students have the knowledge, and are taught the skill, it is only through repeating that skill many times and starting to experience the many differences that occur in wounds and in wound dressings that the student can start to gain an ability to feel confident and be fully independent. Certainly, within this example, it may be very difficult to gain all of this necessary experience during the student's education. It means that, at the point of qualifying, the nurse has the understanding and some ability, but in terms of doing the skill remains a novice requiring experience in different situations (Edmond, 2001).

In very specialist areas, there is an understanding that nurses, regardless of experience, may not have the full range of skills to care fully for the patients they have in that area, for example in an intensive care unit. In specialist units, therefore, there is frequently a well-defined and often extensive supportive induction programme to ensure that nurses feel both confident and competent to work effectively (Cronin and Cronin, 2006). Gaining experience post-qualification needs understanding and acceptance from both the newly qualified nurse and experienced nurses that there needs to be a period in which the newly qualified nurse can settle into the new role and gradually develop their confidence and skills (Clark and Holmes, 2007).

Very specific concerns can include issues that were not able to be practised in great detail during the nurse's preparation programme. This is often due to the local procedures and protocols in an area that does not allow students to be fully independent within the process (for example, medicine administration). Thus there is a perception that students are not allowed to be seen as fully competent until they have become registered nurses, or that they may not necessarily meet particular situations within their nurse preparation programmes (for example, a dying patient).

- **Medicines administration** – Stressful at any stage of the nurse's career, this is particularly stressful for the newly qualified nurse (Gerrish, 2000; O'Shea and Kelly, 2007). On qualifying, some nurses will prefer to continue to check medicines until their confidence increases through good preceptorship.
- **New experiences, for example death of a patient, cardiac arrest** – Occurring after the newly registered nurse qualifies makes it potentially more worrying and difficult to cope

with (Brown and Edelmann, 2000; O'Shea and Kelly, 2007). Whether the situation was experienced during or after training, it is always possible to ask for support and help. There are policies and protocols in every area that the newly qualified nurse will need to follow. One of the hardest aspects in this situation is often how to talk to the patient's relatives. Given the situation, it may be the newly qualified nurse who liaises with relatives. Nurses may need to work through how they deal with the issues on both a professional and a personal level.

Essentially, it is vital to be able to talk to a colleague, ideally one also involved in the situation, who can help you to debrief in relation to the situation.

Leadership, management and supervision

There is a need to identify and understand the issues for others in the team – colleagues, clients, laypeople and professionals within a wide range of contexts. Although the student nurse will have had the chance to take charge of a group of patients, maybe the ward area on a shift in their management allocation, there is a continuing need to develop leadership skills, extending abilities in delegation and supervision, while ensuring professional accountability to their patient or clients, colleagues and themselves.

- **Patient dependency** – Both the dependency and the numbers of patients on a ward are increasing. In comparison with the 2007 survey by the Royal College of Nursing (RCN), the average ratio of 6.9 patients (day-time) and 9.1 patients (night-time) per registered nurse (Ball and Pike, 2007) has increased to 7.9 patients (day-time) and 10.6 patients (night-time) on NHS wards, however this is a similar ratio to that seen in 2005 (Ball and Pike, 2009). The ratio of registered nurse to unregistered nursing staff has decreased with only 60 per cent of nursing staff on duty in the day-time being registered nurses (Ball and Pike, 2009).
- **Accountability and responsibility –** It may be a fear of litigation, or of doing something wrong when prioritising care, but feeling responsible is a normal reaction to the change in circumstance in qualifying and is something to get used to. This will change as people respond differently to the qualified nurse and confidence increases. Managing a situation – Being able to deal with situations effectively, cope with unexpected problems, and manage crises and ethical or cultural issues is essential and at times a significant challenge.

Think back to Activity 6.2 and Jess's experiences. Coping with an emergency requires any nurse to think quickly and prioritise the issues, which is difficult for newly qualified nurses. It is not possible for every student to experience a cardiac arrest in placement, yet, post-qualifying, that nurse may need to assist. Recent developments in nurse education in response to commonly identified skill deficits mean that many newly qualified nurses will have had the chance to practise skills used in emergency situations through participating in scenario-based simulation sessions, but this does not diminish the feelings generated in terms of 'what do I do if . . .?'

- **Managing people –** The newly qualified nurse may want initially to work as part of a team consolidating their practical knowledge and skills, and for that reason some newly qualified nurses opt to work in areas where the teamwork culture is absolutely vital in providing the essential care, for example in emergency departments (Cronin and Cronin, 2006). Other nurses prefer to work in more general areas, both within a hospital or in the community. If the newly qualified nurse is responsible for their group of patients, possibly with a healthcare support worker (HCSW), they may need to delegate and organise care. Delegation is a skill that can require a lot of diplomacy and tact, particularly if they are feeling less confident and if the HCSW is very experienced. It may be, too, that the usual routine that the HCSW is used to in that area differs from the care the newly qualified nurse is expecting to give. Awkward situations can occur and the newly qualified nurse may need to think through how they will deal with these, should they occur.

- **Teaching students** – Formally mentoring a student requires the nurse to have consolidated their training to undertake a mentorship course. It may be, though, that the newly qualified nurse's preceptor may also have a student to mentor. As a result, the newly qualified nurse may be asked to work with a student nurse for a shift. Managing students can be very difficult. Gaining confidence in the new role is challenging, without additional stress from someone watching your every move. It can also feel as though the nurse is short-changing the student in that the knowledge and skills they want to teach in a meaningful way are unable to be taught. For the student, though, it may be very different. They may be happier to work with a newly qualified nurse, who they feel understands their position and what it is they need to learn.

It can be daunting, though, to have a student nurse in the team that the newly qualified nurse is in charge of, even if the student is working with their mentor in that team. As in delegating to any person in the team, the newly qualified nurse will want the task they've delegated to be done with understanding and an awareness of the patient's or client's needs. They want it to be done accurately, correctly and well. They therefore need to be able to trust the person they delegate to. Not jumping in to take over can be very difficult and yet may be something they do need to do. Mentoring students is a difficult and much underrated task at times.

Not all students necessarily are enthusiastic and wanting to learn. Supporting the weaker student is difficult and is outside the scope of this chapter.

Quality and service development

Newly qualified nurses also need to understand the politics of the organisation as it affects them, their patients or clients and their colleagues, so it can be very useful to look at, and be informed about, the strategic view of the organisation they are working in.

It is important to look at the quality of the nursing care that is given to patients to ensure it is effective, efficient, timely and relevant to the needs of the patient at that point in time, but that can feel frustrating and be difficult to achieve when there are time restraints and work piles up (Maben et al., 2007). The nurse will also need to consider the quality of care that the others in that team are providing, for example HCSW or allocated student nurse. If newly qualified nurses identify idiosyncrasies, they need to be able to report these to the appropriate person, often the ward sister or the unit/department manager. There may be explanations that are acceptable for the issues in question; however, the newly qualified nurse may also be identifying a problem that needs addressing. It can often be easier to see the issues as a new person, unused to the area. The newly qualified nurse needs to feel confident enough to identify and report problems, but this can be extremely difficult to do in practice.

Activity 6.4   *Critical thinking*

Read through the following two situations. Which would you rather be in, if you had to be, and why?

It's your third day on a general medical ward. You find your preceptor has rung in sick (half an hour ago). There are two other staff nurses (one in charge) and two HCSWs on the shift with you. The nurse in charge rings her superior for support, only to be told that the directorate is very stretched and no one is currently available, but if possible somebody will be sent.

Situation A

Very apologetically, the nurse in charge asks if you would mind taking the seven patients you had yesterday evening and an extra five patients this morning. She asks the more experienced of the HCSWs to work with you. The other staff nurse and HCSW take the other 13 patients on the ward.

You walk around your patients to identify your priorities and say hello. You ascertain that a number of them require medication with their breakfast (something you remain very nervous about), two need help to sort themselves out before they can eat and three have intravenous infusions that need monitoring.

Situation B

You are allocated with the other staff nurse to care for 12 patients between you. The other team is being run by the nurse in charge with two HCSWs. As a result of the skill differences, your team has the patients on intravenous infusions to care for, while the other team has the patients requiring more basic care with their 'activities of living' (see pages 81–2 in Chapter 4).

The experienced staff nurse recognises that you need to develop confidence, so asks if you would like to be the person in charge, using her as your second person. You agree. Together, you both walk around the patients to identify your priorities and say hello. You ascertain that a number of the patients require medication with their breakfast, one needs help before being able to eat and nine have intravenous infusions that need monitoring.

- Reflect on how these two scenarios differ.
- How would you prioritise the care required and what would you delegate within your team?
- How would you feel about being a part of either team if you were working on this shift? What issues are you concerned about?
- In the area in which you are currently working, talk to your experienced colleagues. How did they feel about their first few days of doing the job they're currently doing?
- Did they feel a need to show they could be independent and capable?

continued opposite . . .

continued . . . •••

- Were they able to ask for help easily without potentially feeling this was a sign of not being able to do the job?

An outline answer is given at the end of the chapter.

Education, training and development

Being aware of your limitations and knowing when to seek support is essential to becoming an independent and confident practitioner (Pratt, 2001). As a student nurse, there will usually have been issues that needed to be researched and analysed. This experience, albeit very academic, provides the newly qualified nurse with an ability to start to look at more practical problems in the clinical area.

All nurses should expect to keep on learning. This may not be through undertaking a course, but in extending knowledge and skills in practice as they gain in experience. The need to understand the issues for a specific patient in order to support and manage the care of that patient may mean looking at current research and the evidence base in order to be able to use relevant information in discussions, thus being an effective advocate for the patient (Cronin and Cronin, 2006).

Nurses need to continue to be reflective about their nursing practice, managing their own professional development and handling their emotions, as well as building and sustaining professional relationships. They need to maintain and further develop a professional portfolio showing how they both achieved and maintained their professional development and expertise (Bick, 1999). Reflecting on what you know needs to be acknowledged personally and becomes the basis for action planning and further learning (Hardyman and Hickey, 2001). Depending on what is identified, it may be that the ward/area is able to provide opportunities to learn that skill or it may be that the nurse needs to reconsider their preferred area of nursing at this stage of their career.

Expecting and finding support

The following are some of the identified support mechanisms.

- **Preceptorship** – Similar to having a mentor when a student nurse, the preceptor is an experienced nurse on the same part of the nursing register as the newly qualified nurse who can provide guidance, help, advice and support. This supports the newly qualified nurse in integrating into the team, developing professional competency and confidence within their new 'qualified nurse' role (Hardyman and Hickey, 2001; Beecroft et al., 2006; NMC, 2006; Kim, 2007). Essentially, the preceptor will provide objective, honest and positive feedback on the nurse's performance, developing plans to achieve the standards set by the employer (NMC, 2006). The terms 'mentor' and 'preceptor' are confusing in the literature and, at times, are used interchangeably, yet evidence from qualitative research shows development of competent practice and is valued by newly qualified nurses (Amos, 2001; Clark and Holmes, 2007; Cummins, 2008; NMC, 2008a). Current guidance from the NMC (2009) within the UK recommends a mandatory period of around six months' preceptorship for all newly qualified nurses in all areas.

- **Clinical supervision** – Clinical supervision provides a setting where an experienced supervisor can help a nurse or group of nurses work through and understand the issues in a situation they've experienced, providing support and potentially guidance (Bick, 1999; Gass et al., 2007; Cummins, 2008). For the newly qualified nurse, the preceptor often takes on this role.
- **Induction programmes** – These help to introduce the nurse to the hospital and the area they will be working in. In most community areas, acute wards and particularly in specialist or critical care areas, the newly qualified nurse may find a well-established induction programme that allows them to consolidate their knowledge and skills.
- **Rotational posts** – Large acute NHS Trusts often operate a rotational system for the first year to 18 months post-qualifying, where the newly qualified nurse has the chance to develop skills in different areas of nursing before settling in one area of their choice. Usually this system means they would change wards every six months, experiencing medical nursing, surgical nursing and possibly a speciality. This can help to boost confidence post-qualifying.

Activity 6.5   *Reflection*

- Look back at the notes you made in relation to Activities 6.2 and 6.4.
- Think about and make a note of the degree and types of support you think you might need in these situations.
- Where do you think that support might come from?

An outline answer is given at the end of the chapter.

There will be many challenges once you have completed your nurse preparation programme and qualified. Getting through these is not necessarily easy, but it is rewarding and satisfying. Some nurses don't manage to complete their nurse education and, of those that do, some may only stay in nursing a short time – just a few months. Looking at the reasons given in the literature for nurses leaving, there are a number of issues, including those of increased stress and workload (Ball and Pike, 2007). It's important to understand that nurse education and qualifying is not the end of the process, but the start of a fulfilling and challenging, ever changing job.

Finding a job – practical issues

One of the first challenges as the student nurse reaches their management and final placements is to find, apply for and accept a job. The newly qualified nurse may know exactly what area of nursing they want to work in and possibly where they are aiming to be working in five to ten years' time. If they do, they need to think about planning how to get to that point, looking at the skills, knowledge and experience that the ideal job requires, then working towards that goal. If, like most nurses on qualifying, the newly qualified nurse isn't sure, they need to try what they enjoy most and develop their nursing career more gradually.

The criteria for how many students are educated are determined by what the Trusts local to the university request to be trained by the local Health Authority. This is not an exact number, as the turnover of staff can vary in an organisation from year to year. However, in terms of the newly qualified nurse getting their first qualified nursing post, the local Trust will likely have jobs available that the newly qualified nurse can apply for and be interviewed for with their peers. Hopefully, there are enough jobs available for everyone who would like one where they want it. There can be extreme disappointment, though, if the newly qualified nurse is one of the people who does not get the first job they are interviewed for.

In recent years, in the UK, nursing posts have not been as readily available, but as NHS Trusts are redesigning and rationalising their workforces, there is a realisation that high-quality patient care depends to an extent on excellent nursing care. To give him- or herself the best chance of getting that first job, the newly qualified nurse needs to try to be open-minded about what they want to do and where they want to be. Being flexible and able to move around the country can mean the newly qualified nurse gets experience before eventually being more selective about the specific jobs that they want.

Activity 6.6   *Critical thinking*

Read through the case study below, then think about the following questions.

- What would your priorities be in getting that first post?
- What are the important factors for you in working out where you want to be and what you would be happy doing?
- Would you be happy to give up any factors in your lifestyle?

Joe has a wife and one child and wants to work in a coronary care unit close to home, but these jobs are not locally available. What is available, though, is a post in a town 100 miles away on a medical assessment unit. It's difficult, but he takes it – he needs to pay the bills each month. Practically, he can stay in accommodation while he works his shifts, then go home on his days off.

Once he'd worked there for four months, he noticed a job nearer to home on a general medical ward. Although still not coronary care, he now had four months' experience post-qualifying. Being far more confident by having some post-course experience, he got the job. Life became easier.

An outline answer is given at the end of the chapter.

Finding a post

Many posts are advertised in the nursing journals or on nursing websites, for example the NHS jobs website. Individual hospital websites will have web pages that advertise the available jobs. Similarly, Community Trust websites often have locally based jobs advertised on their Human Resources pages, or check the local newspaper, too. For specific jobs in mental health nursing, learning disability and children's nursing, it can be useful to check the specific relevant journals that are published in relation to the area of nursing.

Activity 6.7   *Critical thinking*

- Look at the duties identified in the following general job description.
- What are the issues that you need to think about for a job in your preferred area?

Job details

	Staff Nurse
Grade:	Band 5
Accountable to:	Sister/Charge Nurse/Senior nurse in the area
Department/Ward:	Nightingale Ward/Nightingale Directorate

Job purpose

The staff nurse will manage a defined caseload, using evidence-based practice to plan, deliver and evaluate nursing interventions in a variety of settings for their patients or clients. The staff nurse is expected to work in partnership with patients and clients, parents and relatives, appropriate professional colleagues and agencies to undertake a full range of responsibilities – direct patient care, health promotion and implementation of initiatives to ensure the health needs of the patients or clients are recognised and met.

Duties/key areas of responsibility

- Plan, deliver and evaluate nursing care provided for the patient or client, whether routine (developing individualised care) or complex (involving multiple agencies to support the patient's care).
- Develop practice in the assessment and evaluation of patient care.
- Plan and coordinate specific care programmes.
- Promote a multidisciplinary approach to care, ensuring effective communication is maintained between all staff, patients and their families.
- Be competent in the administration of medications, including the calculation of medicines within the clinical area, following NMC guidelines.
- Apply appropriate communication and interpersonal skills to achieve maximum understanding.

continued opposite . . .

---

continued . . .

- Where English is not the first language or understanding is limited or required in a different mode, interventions should be sought to maximise understanding – for example, translator services or resources for the visually impaired, hearing impaired, etc.
- Adhere to the NMC *Code of Professional Conduct* for nurses, midwives and health visitors. Maintain NMC competency and take opportunities for personal and professional development in your professional role through undertaking appropriate mandatory and supplementary/additional training.
- Develop own and others' knowledge and practice across professional and organisational boundaries.
- Use evidence-based practice to develop and maintain a high standard of care and contribute towards the development of the nursing service in this area.
- Be familiar with the Trust's policies, procedures, protocols and standards.
- Participate in the development of new policies, procedures and standards as required within the ward/department.
- Keep accurate, comprehensive, updated records and written reports.
- Participate in clinical supervision as required.
- Report accidents, incidents and complaints according to agreed Trust procedures.
- Be responsible with other staff and ward managers in maintaining a safe environment for patients, visitors and other staff on the ward/in the department.
- Maintain keyboard skills to support the writing of records and reports in the correct format.
- Other duties are likely to include very specific issues that are required within the post being advertised, for example:
  – developing and planning health promotion initiatives;
  – developing, sustaining and evaluating partnerships between individuals, groups, communities and agencies.

The major issues are identified at the end of the chapter.

Applying for a job

When applying for that first job or subsequent posts, the nurse will need to think about different issues, particularly the following.

- **Cover letter** – Should be a business letter written ideally to a named person, maybe in the personnel department or preferably the matron/senior nurse responsible for the post being advertised. It should be brief and polite, yet positive and honest, and should create a professional image. It needs to state what the nurse has previously done, what qualifications they have/are getting and what post they are applying for.
- **Curriculum vitae (CV)** – If the newly qualified nurse is asked to write a CV, it should be short – ideally one to two pages. It should include what they've done, what they can do, what

they know and the job they would like to have. Where possible, it should be targeted towards what the employer wants. CVs are often written, however, to personnel departments when no job is currently being advertised – the nurse who is about to qualify/newly qualified would like that hospital to be aware of them at the point at which a job becomes available.

- **Application form** – This can be easier to write than a CV – the prompts for each section are usually straightforward – name, qualifications, etc. Don't leave gaps, particularly in employment history – this will be asked about, even if childcare related, or due to unemployment or travelling, etc. The hardest part of filling in the form is often the large space available to write how you would be the best person the employer could have to do the job. Review your notes in Activity 6.7; use the job description as a prompt to ensure everything is covered logically and fluently.

Many posts now have online application forms, which can be filled out more quickly, but make sure to check the spellings and grammar that you use. First impressions are important. Ideally, fill out the form and write a draft supporting statement separately, save it, then check for any errors before finally sending the completed, checked form off via email or letter.

- **References** – These consist of opinions written in relation to how well the referee sees the nurse's abilities and personality to undertake the role applied for. Previous employers will be able to comment on the nurse's past experiences and performance as well as their personality and qualities. For a first nursing post, it is essential to use a reference from the place where the newly qualified nurse undertook their preparation programme. This is likely to summarise their nurse education and may include comments from mentors made during the course. The other reference is likely to be from someone the newly qualified nurse has worked closely with, for example a mentor during one of their last practice placements. Always check that the mentor would be happy to do this, though, as they may need support too, particularly if this is the first reference the mentor has written.

After that first post, the qualified nurse will usually drop the nurse education reference when looking for second or subsequent jobs. The current employer would then be the usual first reference to use. It is essential, when putting referees' names on a CV or application form, to make sure the referee has been asked for their permission. Usually, references will be taken up only after the nurse has been interviewed, although this varies between employers. The qualified nurse may require a nurse education reference after their first job if they plan to undertake another academic course, for example a specialist nursing degree course, when the university may require an academic reference.

The interview

- **Preparation** – Similar to applying, it is important to find out about the job, what the role would demand and the potential employer. Ideally, it is best to go for an informal interview, although this can be difficult if distance is an issue. Pre-interview visits are usually informal, but need to be arranged via the telephone or by letter. Looking at the environment, as well as meeting a few of the staff the nurse may be working with if successful at the interview, can help the nurse to decide if they definitely want this specific job. It can help to ask questions informally and to identify questions to ask formally at the interview.

- **Dress** – Be smart and professional yet comfortable with what you are wearing.
  - Women – Don't wear a top with a revealing cleavage. This can put interviewers off, making them wonder how professional you would be with the patients and clients. Similarly, don't wear jeans – even smart ones. Again, it can create a negative impression.
  - Men – A suit is ideal, but trousers, shirt and tie are fine. The outfit needs to be conservative, though, so don't go for bright colours and patterns. Be neat and professional.
- **Interview questions** – These are usually related to the role, previous experiences, and qualities and abilities required to undertake the job, and may be based on the duties identified in the job description (Activity 6.7). The nterviewer is trying to ensure they appoint the person who is most able to do the job they have, someone who will fit in with the rest of the team and a person who is willing to do the job.
  - Questions vary, but there are recurrent themes. Think about the area and the possible questions that might arise, as follows.
  - Basic understanding of the issues facing qualified nurses – This can include having a working knowledge of clinical supervision, preceptorship, accountability, primary nursing, lifelong learning, patient advocacy, clinical governance, audit and anything specific to the area, such as working with families, Every Child Matters, the Mental Health Act, challenging behaviours, etc.
  - Clinical situations – Questions may include how the interviewee would deal with a specific situation. These are usually fairly general in nature and may require logical thought about what to do, for example if the controlled drug keys were accidentally taken out of the hospital by a member of staff forgetting to hand them over at the end of the shift; or if a patient absconded.
  - Current nursing issues – Questions can also be related to current issues in the media, such as who the current Health Secretary is, particularly if the job you are applying for is high profile in terms of public interest.
  - Personal questions – Why have you chosen this speciality? Have you read any research that you could use in this area/ward? Where do you see yourself in five years' time?
  - General questions – Why are you interested in this job? Tell us about yourself. What are your strengths and weaknesses? How do you relax? What skills can you bring to this job? What do you see as the main challenges to working here?
- **Professional portfolio** – This will be developed throughout nurse education courses and can help to provide evidence of what you've previously done. Prospective employers may not ask for it, but you can always offer it and use it to show your abilities.
- **Presentation** – Although unusual for a first post, the newly qualified nurse may be asked to prepare a topic for discussion or presentation. Always make sure you know exactly what is expected and prepare it comprehensively just as would be done for any academic assignment. This can make the difference between the knowledgeable, motivated, yet inexperienced newly qualified nurse and an experienced nurse who potentially needs to update their knowledge in the area.
- **Equal opportunities** – It is illegal to discriminate in an interview in terms of gender, pregnancy, religion, disability or age. It may be, though, that, as the interviewee, you bring up an issue that would affect your immediate employability, for example pregnancy.

After the interview

Each interview is a chance to get the post and to showcase knowledge and abilities. It is also a place to learn and develop the skills of being interviewed. Getting offered the job is fantastic, while not getting it is upsetting and frustrating. Whatever happens, it is useful to note down the questions that were asked and to ring the employer and ask for interview feedback. Are there issues that the nurse was not aware of – mannerisms, perhaps, or any weak areas, any positive areas? Was there anything that caused confusion? Think about the responses and don't give up. Be prepared and be confident.

The total number of nurses changing jobs – measured as the turnover, in 2007 had dropped significantly to around 16 per cent (Ball and Pike, 2007). In 2009, this has increased to 19 per cent as nurses feel more able to change jobs. As NHS Trusts have restructured their workforce, so the feelings in 2007 of uncertainty and anxieties about redundancy and job losses have stabilised. The 2009 survey identifies that the majority of nurses moving jobs (54 per cent) is as part of early career progression – experiencing other areas of nursing and consolidating skills, although there is movement between jobs relating both to increasing workloads and stress (31 per cent) and dissatisfaction with the previous post (30 per cent) (Ball and Pike, 2009).

How well people work is based on integrating the knowledge and skills they've gained through their training with good preceptorship, access to good support, resources and good working conditions. Having the correct number and skill mix of nurses in the department directly influences the degree of patient satisfaction felt. A shortage of nurses or multidisciplinary staff within the team, poor resources or just a poor skill mix – for example, too many junior nurses – can tip the balance in increasing the workload and the demand on maybe one or two of the team on that shift. That leads to frustration and eventually poor morale within the team. If unchecked, potentially there is a rise in staff sickness and in people, particularly the more skilled and experienced people, leaving the team.

Employment

- **Professional register** – The NMC requires an initial fee for the newly qualified nurse to be registered on the appropriate part of the nursing and midwifery register. This registration is reviewed annually and the nurse will need to state and sign to say they are able to practise as a nurse on a yearly basis. This yearly registration carries a fee to remain on the active nursing register as a registered, practising nurse.
- **Contract of employment** – This is a binding, legal agreement between the employer and the employee. It is a formal, written document that identifies exactly what the nurse is expected to do within the job he or she is appointed to. The nurse will be expected to sign this on taking up employment. It can comprise either one or a number of documents, as follows.
- **Job description** – This identifies the expectations of the nurse by their employer within the role. It will identify the hours of work they are expected to undertake within the job, the date of commencement of the post, and starting salary, This will often also identify the managerial structure that the nurse reports to and who oversees what the nurse does from the employer perspective.

- **Person specification** – This details the requirements the post-holder needs.
- **Knowledge and Skills Framework (KSF) document** – In the UK NHS, this document details the knowledge requirements of the post. This can support the post-holder's individual learning and provide an ongoing framework to review the post-holder's progress.
- **Terms of employment** – In large organisations, for example the NHS, this is often a standard document, so may be separate; however, it forms part of the employment contract identifying the employee's rights to benefits, such as annual leave entitlement and maternity benefits, as well as identifying procedures for absence, sickness protocols, disciplinary procedure, redundancy, grievances, etc.
- **Ongoing/lifelong learning** – It is important periodically to review your learning and action planning. Within a specific job in the NHS, the KSF can support the development of knowledge and skills required to undertake the job the postholder is doing. As the nurse becomes more experienced following their initial registration, there will be opportunities to extend skills and abilities – maybe through giving intravenous medication or cannulation.

The pace of learning often slows. The way forward is through reflection on practice – keeping a professional portfolio of the issues arising and potential incidents that you learn from and potentially use anonymously to discuss with your preceptor or close colleagues. Clinical supervision is used differently in different areas with varying levels of success, but as a professional environment in which to share experiences and work through tension and emotions, it can be essential in making sense of a critical incident that occurred, perhaps in looking at the way care is provided or in exploring other ways of dealing with a specific situation.

Finance – wages and pay

Registered nurses made up around 60 per cent of nursing staff in the NHS in 2009; 64 per cent in independent hospital wards and 25 per cent in care homes (Ball and Pike, 2009). There is a continuing difference between specialities, in that registered nurses account for about 48 per cent of nursing staff on wards for older people, 62 per cent on general adult wards, 50 per cent on mental health wards and 83 per cent on paediatric wards (Ball and Pike, 2009).

NHS sector – In 2005–6, the way NHS professionals in the UK were paid changed to a system called Agenda for Change. As a result of the change, each job in the NHS was assessed and regraded to provide 'equal pay for equal work' within all grades of staff (excluding medical staff). This has a total of nine grades within it, although band 8 has four parts – a, b, c and d. The majority of nurses are graded as bands 5 and 6, with ward sisters and some community nurses on band 7. The only nurses in band 8, usually 8a, are those who are matrons or who have increased clinical responsibilities as consultant nurses or nurse practitioners.

It is the job that is graded, not the person, so whether the newly qualified nurse has completed a basic nursing course or has a Master's in Nursing, as a newly qualified person, it is their registration as a nurse that counts. Each role is assessed in relation to the job description and carries with it the wage the nurse can expect in undertaking that role. As the nurse progresses through their career, their academic qualification(s) will be taken more into consideration depending on the role then being undertaken; for example, specialist nurses often have a Master's degree or are working towards an advanced qualification. This can potentially increase the band at which they are paid.

In the UK banding system, newly qualified nurses are paid on the band 5 scale. Wages will increase for every full year of work, going up in increments on each scale until the ceiling for that band is reached, or until the nurse is required to show ongoing professional development in terms of knowledge and skills to get to the next part of the same band. If the nurse works part-time, then the increase is dependent on them reaching the equivalent of one year's work full time.

- **Private sector** – In the UK, nurses in the private sector may not be paid under the Agenda for Change rules, but tend to be paid around the same level as the equivalent nurse within the NHS system. As such, it means the nurse can opt in or out of the private sector to gain experience when desired. There may also be other incentives, possibly financial or annual leave entitlements, etc., that are slightly different but that suit the nurse and their circumstances better than those in the NHS.
- **Working abroad** – Wages will be similar to those in the UK for the same role in other countries. The nurse's standard of living, though, can change and working abroad is totally dependent on a number of factors, of which the wage is only one aspect to consider.
- **Getting paid** – There will be changes in the next few years in relation to all nurses undertaking a degree course in order to become a registered nurse. Currently, though, there are still a few Diploma level courses but this is being phased out nationally in the UK. Studying on a Diploma course means that the student can access a non-means-tested bursary to support their studies; however, that bursary is likely to become means-tested for the degree studies.

If the student does get a bursary, then this is often paid at the beginning of the month, whereas wages tend to be paid in arrears, so at the end of the month. In addition, the initial bursary paid to the student may be a double amount, so there is a need to budget well in order to ensure bills can be paid during the transfer from student to staff nurse, which may mean a gap of at least eight weeks between these two payments.

Coping with the money can be difficult to do and financial advice is always worth seeking. There will be advisers who can help you via the Student Union as part of the University while you are a student.

Once you have the job as a newly qualified nurse, you will need to think through issues around Christmas particularly. The monthly payment is usually the week before Christmas in most NHS Trusts, leaving you with six to seven weeks to cope with the post-Christmas bills before you're paid again!

- **What's it like coping with the money?** – Entering the workforce means starting to develop another stage of life. Whether the nurse chooses to settle down or further their professional or academic experiences, a regular income is essential to ensure they can live, work and play more easily, possibly, than before. The nurse can apply for and obtain a mortgage or start to pay off any debts incurred as a student.
- **Deductions** – On getting a wage slip, there are a number of deductions made prior to being paid. This needs to be understood as it details how the wage the nurse gets is calculated and the how the take-home pay is worked out. Legally, all employees have a right to an itemised statement of their pay at the time of, or just prior to, being paid. If the employee doesn't understand any part of it, they can ask the finance department or employer to clarify any confusion.

Wage slip	
Gross pay (amount before deductions)	**Tax code** (usually a letter and a number)
Deductions: National insurance contribution Income tax Pension contributions	**Personally arranged deductions**: e.g. Trade union subscription Childcare payment
Final pay (after all the deductions) – this is the amount you have to use until the next pay day!	

- **National Insurance (UK payment)** – These are payments made by the employee that entitle them to social security benefits, for example incapacity benefit or unemployment benefit. Depending on pension arrangements, the employee may pay a different rate of National Insurance from that paid by colleagues. National Insurance is also paid by your employer to the Government.
- **Tax** – Each person working in the UK is entitled to a personal allowance that is reviewed each year in the Budget. Once the employee's total income exceeds the personal allowance threshold, the employee will be expected to pay tax on earnings above the threshold amount.
- **Pensions** – Every employee should think about paying something towards the need for finance when they retire. It is possible to opt out of the superannuation NHS pension scheme; however, as with everyone not employed in the NHS, it is important both to think about and to ensure you start paying something each month into a reputable pension scheme.
- **Joining a trade union** – It is also important to think about joining a trade union. Joining can provide the employee with legal advice and free assistance if there are work-related issues, such as accidents, and can provide legal support and protection from discrimination.
- **Joining a professional organisation** – Joining an organisation that relates professionally to your preferred area can be useful for resources, advice and relevant information.

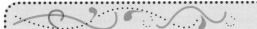

Chapter summary

Patients and clients deserve and require the best nurses. Being a qualified nurse, and helping, supporting and caring for patients and clients of all ages is at times challenging, at times frustrating. Yet it is both enjoyable and satisfying. Patients and clients will expect a newly qualified nurse to be clinically competent; however, this should not be confused with a possible lack of confidence when starting in a new clinical area. Newly qualified nurses need to give themselves time to develop, while ensuring that what they are doing is done using their skills of reflection and critical thinking, and ensuring that their patients receive the best care they can give in a timely way, integrating knowledge and clinical skills using the best available evidence. Above all, newly qualified nurses need to be aware of their limitations. Issues, incidents and problems need to be discussed, maybe with a preceptor, a senior colleague or through clinical supervision.

continued overleaf . . .

continued . . . •••

Think through the opportunities that are there. Newly qualified nurses need to think about what they want and where they see themselves being within nursing. There are lots of people working with you, working within the same organisation or working outside the organisation – in a trade union or professional support role – to ask for advice. Planning your career is essential, and becoming a newly qualified nurse is just the beginning of what can be a very satisfying and rewarding career choice.

Activities: brief outline answers

Activity 6.1 (page 120)

You may have identified issues in relation to dexterity, such as coordinating different parts of the body, for example mind, breathing and limbs when trying to swim using breaststroke; or coordinating your foot on the accelerator pedal with the clutch in setting off on a 'hill start' when driving a car.

Feeling scared is a common feeling among most of us when we start anything new; it is very possible that you identified feelings of nervousness, even fear, yet also probably feelings of elation and satisfaction when you mastered the skill.

Activity 6.2 (pages 121–2)

Jess is obviously a competent nurse who has achieved well academically and who is completing her competences prior to qualifying. She's still learning, though, developing her management skills and her confidence in rapidly changing situations. Like Jess, you may have identified issues relating to feeling underconfident and in reacting to situations rather than being able to think effectively through situations.

This is challenging, but priorities can be identified. Using management techniques, such as delegation, is essential to keeping an overview of the situation. Knowing the skills and abilities of who you are working with means you can effectively oversee and control potentially very difficult situations.

Activity 6.4 (pages 128–9)

In the first scenario, you may feel very alone and responsible for the total care of patients in the team. The second scenario potentially provides more reassurance and confidence, although the patient dependency is possibly higher. In terms of giving medications, it is probably easier to seek support in the second scenario than in the first, where you would need to ask the nurse in charge for help, which may take him or her away from important managerial issues.

Prioritising care is easier in the second one – intravenous infusions need reading hourly, and those patients may need support with hygiene and dressing, as does the patient needing help prior to breakfast. Potentially, delegating the medication to the experienced staff will allow you to support the patient requiring help prior to breakfast. While this means you may not be learning as this medication is given, it addresses the priorities of care. Given the number of intravenous infusions and potentially more medications later on, you won't lose out in relation to learning opportunities.

Both scenarios can and do happen.

Activity 6.5 (page 130)

In Activity 6.4, support would come from the others on the ward, while in 6.2 it is very much from Jess's mentor. As such, you may have identified a need for preceptorship or just someone to talk the issue through with. Immediate support is usually available from colleagues, but support can be wider, including counselling within the organisation and potentially also outside agencies, too, for example advisory groups in a professional forum. Not all support is accessible at the time you need it, which can be an issue.

Activity 6.6 (page 131)

Your priorities may be very specific, but you may have looked at, or need to think about, a number of factors in finding your ideal job.

- What if it's not available at the moment?
- What job would you like to be doing – what post would be ideal for you?
- Where would you like to be working?
- How can you develop experiences to enable you to become a 'good' candidate and give yourself the best chance of getting that ideal job?
- It's essential to think about developing your career in nursing, not jumping from one job to another as you feel like it.

Activity 6.7 (pages 132–3)

Within this activity you need to think specifically about your current abilities in relation to the duties of the job you are applying for. This particular job description has very general duties identified that are common to most job descriptions, and there may be many other key responsibilities identified. There may also be specific issues for you to consider, depending on your area of nursing, for example:

- adult nursing;
- mental health nursing;
- children's nursing;
- learning disability nursing;
- midwifery.

You also need to think how you would provide evidence of being able to develop practice, in order to plan and coordinate care. One way is to develop a professional portfolio, which helps to highlight and provide evidence of what you've done previously.

Taking it to your interview would be ideal and you may decide to use post-it notes on the sections that specifically pertain to issues in the job description.

For example, if you have previously introduced an initiative into the area you are working in, you could use it as an illustration in the interview and indicate the evidence in your accompanying portfolio. As a student nurse, you may have dealt very effectively with a critical incident and then reflected on the situation with your mentor. You could provide the witness statement or a reflection within your portfolio.

The personal statement on the application form needs to address what you can provide in terms of the duties required in this post. That can then be supported with the professional portfolio that you take to the interview.

Further reading

For details on the Agenda for Change and the KSF, see**: Department of Health (DH)** (2004) *The NHS Knowledge and Skills Framework (NHS KSF) and the Development Review Process.* Available online at **www.dh. gov.uk/en/Publicationsandstatistics/Publications/PublicationsPolicyAndGuidance/DH_ 4090843**

Department of Health (DH) (2004) *Agenda for Change.* Available online at **www.dh.gov.uk/ en/Managingyourorganisation/Humanresourcesandtraining/Modernisingpay/Agenda forchange/DH_424**.

Useful websites

www.dh.gov.uk/en/Publicationsandstatistics

Here you can find a copy of *Modernising Nursing Careers.*

www.hmrc.gov.uk

Look under the 'individuals and employees' section for information on tax, national insurance and childcare support. This is a useful introduction to the subject.

www.jobs.nhs.uk

This is the NHS Jobs website.

www.nmc-uk.org.uk

The site of the Nursing and Midwifery Council (NMC).

www.rcm.org.uk

The site of the Royal College of Midwives.

www.rcn.org.uk/support/pay_and_conditions/agendaforchange

Contains details of the Agenda for Change and other information on pay and conditions.

www.worksmart.org.uk

This is the Worksmart website of the Trades Union Congress (TUC).

Chapter 7
Exploring the world of nursing by those working in it

Carol Hall, with Liz Aston and colleagues,
Justine Barksby, Karen Billyeald,
Louise Cook, Paula Dawson, Anne Felton,
Bob Hallawell, Sheila Rose, Helen Saxelby,
Gemma Stacey and Theo Stickley

NMC Standards for Pre-registration Nursing Education

This chapter echoes Chapter 1 by using the generic standards for competence for all four fields of practice to set a benchmark for how nursing should be. The content of the interviews that follow should be seen in the context of these generic standards.

Domain 1: Professional values

All nurses must act first and foremost to care for and safeguard the public. They must practise autonomously and be responsible and accountable for safe, compassionate, person-centred, evidence-based nursing that respects and maintains dignity and human rights. They must show professionalism and integrity and work within recognised professional, ethical and legal frameworks. They must work in partnership with other health and social care professionals and agencies, service users, their carers and families in all settings, including the community, ensuring that decisions about care are shared.

Domain 2: Communication and interpersonal skills

All nurses must use excellent communication and interpersonal skills. Their communications must always be safe, effective, compassionate and respectful. They must communicate effectively using a wide range of strategies and interventions including the effective use of communication technologies. Where people have a disability, nurses must be able to work with service users and others to obtain the information needed to make reasonable adjustments that promote optimum health and enable equal access to services.

continued overleaf . . .

continued . . .

Domain 3: Nursing practice and decision making

All nurses must practise autonomously, compassionately, skilfully and safely, and must maintain dignity and promote health and wellbeing. They must assess and meet the full range of essential physical and mental health needs of people of all ages who come into their care. Where necessary they must be able to provide safe and effective immediate care to all people prior to accessing or referring to specialist services irrespective of their field of practice. All nurses must also meet more complex and coexisting needs for people in their own nursing field of practice, in any setting including hospital, community and at home. All practice should be informed by the best available evidence and comply with local and national guidelines. Decision making must be shared with service users, carers and families and informed by critical analysis of a full range of possible interventions, including the use of up-to-date technology. All nurses must also understand how behaviour, culture, socio-economic and other factors, in the care environment and its location, can affect health, illness, health outcomes and public health priorities and take this into account in planning and delivering care.

Domain 4: Leadership, management and team working

All nurses must be professionally accountable and use clinical governance processes to maintain and improve nursing practice and standards of healthcare. They must be able to respond autonomously and confidently to planned and uncertain situations, managing themselves and others effectively. They must create and maximise opportunities to improve services. They must also demonstrate the potential to develop further management and leadership skills during their period of preceptorship and beyond.

Chapter aims

After reading this chapter, you will be able to:

- understand what the nature of practical nursing is, as it is applied to the different fields of qualified nursing practice in the UK;
- see through the eyes of qualified nurses in the field of practice in which you are interested;
- identify experiences you may wish to explore further in your nursing course or in your work;
- make choices about your own future career.

Introduction

In this final part of the book, we present excerpts from group interviews with nurses from each of the main fields of practice of nursing operating in the UK – learning disability, children's, mental health and adult nursing. The nurses talking in the interviews currently work in a range of nursing careers within these fields of practice.

The aim of the chapter is to help you understand the roles and work of these nurses and to explore, from their perspective, what it is like to be a qualified nurse today. It is not intended that the sections will cover every element of nursing practice in each field; indeed, that would be impossible to achieve. However, the aim is to address some key and representative elements of practice and give a flavour of the values and concerns of the profession.

The chapter is divided into the four sections relating to the fields of practice. In each field of practice section, key excerpts and case studies from the interviews are offered as an illustration of the roles and practice of nursing as seen by the nurses interviewed. These are interspersed with discussion, practical activities and opportunities to reflect on the examples given. The excerpts refer to questions set by the interviewer, which asked about the following.

- What is nursing practice in your field, and what skills are needed?
- What are the best parts of working as a nurse and what challenges are there?
- What about the practicalities – what kinds of work can you do?
- Do you have a vision for the future of nursing?

Each field of practice stands alone and can be read in this way, although they all follow a similar format. You can dip into just the field of your own interest or read about as many as you wish. Even if you know which field of nursing you are especially interested in, the issues raised in each section may sometimes be applied to different fields. For example, in children's nursing, the nurses have focused on practices relating to the management of professional relationships. These aspects have application in the different branches to a greater or lesser extent and the thinking behind the discussion may be of interest to others. Finally, you will notice at the end of this chapter that there is a list of all the nurses interviewed, to whom we give our thanks.

It is critical to recognise that the chapter is the work of these practitioners. The insights they were able to offer have made the chapter what it is and I am not only extremely grateful for their willingness to participate, but very much richer in my own understanding about nursing.

What is learning disability nursing?

Concept summary

People with learning disabilities often have a wide range of physical and mental health conditions. Learning disability nurses work in partnership with them and family carers, to provide specialist healthcare. Their main aim is to support the well-being and social inclusion of people with a learning disability by improving or maintaining their physical and mental health, by reducing barriers and by supporting them to pursue a fulfilling life. For example, teaching someone the skills to find work can be significant in helping them to lead a more independent, healthy life where they can relate to others on equal terms. Learning disability nursing is provided in settings such as adult education, residential and community centres, as well as in patients' homes, workplaces and schools. You could specialise in such areas as education, sensory disability or the management of services. If you work in a residential setting, you may do shifts to provide 24-hour care (**www.nhscareers.nhs.uk**).

What is nursing practice in the learning disability field and what skills are needed?

The nurses who participated in the interview were from a range of different areas of learning disability nursing practice and from nursing education. In the first excerpt they talk about the variety and range of roles and practices that they undertake in working with people with special learning needs.

Activity 7.1   *Reflection*

Before you read LD Excerpt 1, try to think of the types of work that nurses working with clients with learning disabilities might do. Jot down your ideas and save them.

Now read the excerpt and think about the following questions.

- How was learning disability nursing defined by the nurses and what features were identified as important?
- Look at your own notes. Was the way the nurses described their practice something that you expected or did it surprise you at all?

Outline answers are given at the end of the chapter.

LD Excerpt 1

Interviewer: What is nursing practice in learning disability field of practice?

We work everything from child hospices up to high secure forensic (services). We work across a huge spectrum.

We assess and plan and treat like in other fields, but I think we're, in my opinion, we're more diverse . . .

continued opposite . . .

continued . . .

Physical health . . .

Psychological health . . .

And a lot of people in our service also have mental illness, and often we have developmental stuff even if we're not in children's services because of their developmental age . . .

There's a lot about carers and relationships external to the actual individual that we're caring for.

I think so, it's a person-centred kind of approach, but it's a family-centred approach as well.

I think the learning disability nurse becomes the coordinator often, the facilitator of all those different agencies and key players that are involved . . . And the patient or the client is at the centre of that, but there's so much more that feeds into it.

. . . Thinking also about demographic change, the projections are that our work will be much more spread across the lifespan than it potentially has previously. Particularly the older end of the lifespan, where we previously may have had a client group that was prone to die younger than other members of the population; we're not seeing that now, we're seeing people developing the conditions of old age, of the older person that we wouldn't have otherwise experienced. But we're also seeing very more complex children coming through at the other end of the system as well . . .

. . . who previously probably wouldn't have survived

. . . and who (will) potentially come into adult learning disability services later on in their lives. And, as we were saying earlier, the physical healthcare skill is becoming an important agenda for us, I think, in terms of the range of skills, competences, that the learning disabilities nurse needs to possess.

It is clear that to care for such a wide range of individuals, some specific skills are needed. In LD Excerpt 2 the nurses discuss what skills they consider to be most important to them in their work.

LD Excerpt 2

Interviewer: What specific skills do you think are really important; things that you should learn as a student nurse in caring for people with a learning disability?

I think you need communication, communication, communication, definitely.

On all levels . . .

continued overleaf . . .

continued . . . ••

Regardless of where within the speciality you go, communication underpins. But then there's that whole physical side . . . and the really complex physical needs and everything that goes with that whether it's PEG [percutaneous endogastric] feeding, or whatever.

Epilepsy is a huge area in learning disabilities, and being able to have a really sound knowledge base about that, and know what to do. But then there's the whole challenging behaviour side, and the violence and aggression, and being able to deal with that and keep your calm and be cool.

. . . there's a lot of personal management skills in there, aren't there, really as well?

It's also about the psychological side of it as well. I think there's more and more acknowledgement that people with a learning disability can have psychological problems, whereas before it was simply put down to the fact that they had a learning disability. This behaviour was because they were learning disabled. And there's now much more acceptance that actually they have the same emotional and psychological problems as anybody else . . . So learning disability nurses have got to have the skills in actually being able to recognise and know how to treat and manage those situations.

I think there's all this stuff around, you know, safeguarding, and risk assessment, and it's that skill that you develop about making sound judgements *with* people, not *for* people.

You need to be able to think on your feet, I think, in learning disabilities . . .

. . . there is never a dull moment, it's really exciting.

One of the definitions I've heard in the past is about the professional and what makes a professional a professional. One of the definitions is about the capacity to deal with uncertainty and complexity, and that's what differentiates the professional from other members of the health or social care workforce. And I think that's very true of our nurses now in terms of the range of areas that they're being expected to work in and the range of skills that they're being expected to apply in the work that they're actually doing. We've got that sort of huge physical healthcare skill range, we've got the legislative stuff that people have to have a high level of familiarity with and be able to apply, we've got the communication stuff, we've got the psychological stuff, you know, the social development issues. And they're all part of the role in different ways; the more we work as individuals within the community systems, supporting people, the more that range of complex skill is going to be a necessity in the way that people work.

In the above excerpt the nurses talked about the importance of communication, and the capacity to care for very specific physical needs of clients, using the example of administering PEG feeds as one example of a clinical skill required by the nurse. Of course, there are many more such skills that must be learned while becoming a nurse in the learning disability field of practice. The nurses also identify the skill of the nurse in being able to assess complex situations, suggesting that they must be able to determine relative relationships between physical needs, developmental learning ability and disability, and any concurrent psychological and emotional needs. This takes careful assessment and an understanding about the clients with whom you are working, in order to optimise the care of individuals. The nurses also discuss a definition of a professional and what this might mean to their practice.

Activity 7.2 *Critical thinking*

Taking the above discussion about being a professional into account, it is useful to return to Chapter 2 of this book, which addresses the characteristics of the nurse as a professional.

- Compare the short description given by the learning disability nurse with what you read in Chapter 2.
- Now think about everything else that is said by the learning disability nurses in this chapter. Reflect on how many other ways the learning disability nurse can be identified as a professional.

As this activity is based on your own reflection, there is no outline answer at the end of the chapter.

What are the best parts of working as a nurse in learning disability practice and what challenges are there?

In this discussion, learning disability nurses were clear that making differences to their clients' lives was the best part of their roles in many ways, but they also found this challenging, too. They liked the variety and spontaneity of their work in practice and suggested that no two days were the same for them. In LD Excerpt 3, the nurse talks about how performing nursing can empower clients and enable them to participate at different levels in their care. A further example is given in the following case study. Here the nurse recalls a very personally satisfying experience felt during the long-term care of a patient.

LD Excerpt 3

Interviewer: What are the best parts of working as a nurse in learning disability practice?

Just making a difference. Just having somebody who comes to you in a situation where they might be unhappy, unwell . . . you know, to then be able to move them through a process, and . . . we've got person-centred planning tools that are now absolutely out of this world, and if everybody signs up to that way of working it reaps tremendous rewards. To people actually having a life. I'm working with people with learning disabilities now who sit on partnership boards, and who have a stake in developing services, and who are quite happy to say if they're not happy about something and things aren't right. Woe betide you if you don't get things right for them. And that's just fantastic, that's very different to when I came into the profession 20-odd years ago.

continued overleaf . . .

Case study

'I can remember, a few years ago, I worked with a gentleman who had chosen not to communicate verbally for years. He could and he had done in the past but he chose not to. And I worked with him for a few years and then this one particular day he just came up to me and he said 'are you all right then?' and he kissed me on the cheek! And everyone just said 'Wow!', because he'd not verbally spoken for years and years and years, and everyone was talking about it for months after. And just something that small was a major breakthrough with that guy and from that point on he started to speak very slowly but surely and that was just amazing – that was an amazing thing.'

In the following discussion, the nurses talked about what they found challenging in their roles in practice. Two key challenges emerged, the first related to the concept discussed above of achieving within a long-term time-span. The nurses identified that, while this could be one of the best parts of being a learning disability nurse, it could also be very challenging to work with such long-term goals, as you had to persevere. The need to persevere and keep on persevering was recognised as challenging, but ultimately could be rewarding. The second challenge related to the nurses' role in advocating for their patients. While they considered that it was imperative that they were able to empower their patients, the role of the nurse as an advocate was viewed as challenging. LD Excerpt 4 explains this more.

LD Excerpt 4

Interviewer: What are the challenges of being a learning disability nurse?

It [the role of the nurse] is very much about putting the patient, the client, at the centre of what you're doing or trying to do. I mean we have advocacy services but the biggest advocates I've ever seen for people with a learning disability are the nurses.

They will speak up!

Loudly!

And that's one of our challenges, that's always been one of our biggest challenges . . .

The position of people with learning disabilities in our society as a marginalised group, the role of the disability nurse in helping to address that . . .

Championing . . .

To change – that is a challenge.

The nurses address the role of the nurse in advocating for their clients and identify that advocating for their clients is not always easy. They also identify their clients as being a marginalised or disadvantaged group. This is supported by MENCAP in their two hard-hitting and shocking reports – *Treat Me Right* (2004) and *Death By Indifference* (2008). It is important to read the summaries of these reports as they have major implications for nursing. They highlight the need for nurses to pay special attention to those with learning disability who have health needs and the need for nurses to empower and advocate within this profession.

Advocacy is an important concept in nursing and, as shown in Chapter 1 of this book, is identified internationally by the ICN within its definition of nursing. However, the concept of what it means practically to advocate in nursing remains debated.

Activity 7.3   *Research and critical thinking*

Read MacDonald, H (2007) Relational ethics and advocacy in nursing: literature review. *Journal of Advanced Nursing*, 57(2): 119–26.

In this paper you will find that 'advocacy' is defined and, according to MacDonald, it is important to note that:

> *Advocacy in nursing is recognized as a worthy activity and, according to professional codes of ethics, a moral imperative.*
> (p125)

However, the paper also identifies that the actual practice of advocacy is more difficult to define. Consider the research reviewed in this paper and think about the context in which learning disability nurses describe their roles in advocacy. Also return to the considerations of advocacy outlined in Chapters 1 and 2 of this book.

Can you identify any situations in the excerpts so far where the nurse's role in advocating for people with learning disabilities may be difficult or challenged?

A brief outline answer is given at the end of the chapter.

What about the practicalities – what kinds of work can you do?

In this section, the learning disability nurses identify places to work as a qualified nurse. Because the care of learning disabled people varies in definition nationally and globally, jobs may be found in both health and social care settings. In their discussion, however, the value of learning disability nursing as a profession was reiterated by the group and the roles played were clearly identified. For new nurses coming into practice in this area of care, it was identified that a wide appreciation of the work that could be undertaken was necessary, and that looking for work meant looking at jobs that may not necessarily be identified specifically or solely for learning disability nurses. The nurses identified that the broadness of their role meant that developing professionally after qualification had considerable opportunity and huge variety.

Activity 7.4	*Research and evidence-based practice*

The nurses recognised the British Institute of Learning Disabilities as a useful resource for them, with relevant publications and conferences for practitioners.

Take a look at their website on **www.bild.org.uk**.

As this activity is based on your own observations, there is no outline answer at the end of the chapter.

The interviewees emphasised also that the distinction between working in private and public sector care has changed over recent years and that they find many opportunities for learning disability nurses in private and public sector care facilities in the UK.

LD Excerpt 5 continues this discussion.

LD Excerpt 5

Interviewer: What career opportunities are available on qualification?

Often residential in my experience . . .

. . . but even that word, it's massive, because within residential care for people with learning disabilities, there's still NHS provision, then there's loads of private provision and social care, and when I qualified anyone who went into the private sector, you kind of went "really?!" But now there's some fantastic private-sector provision that's going on. That's really doing some really innovative, creative and really good practices. And so that's great for them, and they're working as nurses within private providers. Then there's forensics, which you'll tell us about [laughs].

All different levels of secure services, you've got high, medium, low, and community forensic work that they go into and also the prisons, they can work in the prisons, and as you say they can work in places like hospices, they can be like liaison nurses, like Accident and Emergency care and on to the (hospital) ward . . .

There's a lot of assessment and treatment teams again in very different guises, like the one you were talking about; we've got community assessment and treatment teams here locally as well. But also there's still assessment and treatment units that people go in for a fixed period of time and then come out again. Community nurses again, like we were saying, it used to be a bit more of a senior role, but they're going in at band 5 [newly qualified nurses]. We have day service provision in both health and social services; we've had some recently newly qualified people working as school nurses in special schools . . .

What is the future vision for learning disability nursing?

In a final discussion, the nurses were asked about changes and visions they had for their service. They were clear that a future role in empowering their service users was important, but they also identified the importance of community education in enabling our society to respond to people with learning disabilities in a more inclusive way. They also identified a need for people with learning disabilities to be enabled to become part of local communities.

The following case study illustrates how practitioners challenged assumptions to create changes for their area of learning disability nursing practice.

Case study

'I think the other thing that we do is that we challenge assumptions. And maybe an example of that would be in terms of our assessment and treatment service. It was a bed-based service up to four years ago when the hospital that those beds were within closed. Now, four years later, it has no beds whatsoever. It has access to beds via mental health services, but actually operates as an outreach service. And that has changed the whole philosophy of the way that team works; they've embraced person-centred planning wholeheartedly, and yes there are still a couple of people for whom that doesn't work and you have to sort of acknowledge and accept that, but for the bulk of people it has encouraged them to be far more a part of their communities and the work's been very proactive and very positive, and just sort of trying to get more understanding of why people were behaving in the way that they were behaving, what needs to be there to support them in order for their communities to accept them.'

Conclusion

Learning disability nursing is a diverse and rapidly evolving field of practice in which nurses can really make a difference to the lives of their clients. Learning disability nurses are now working within the three-year strategy (2009–12) from the Department of Health called *Valuing People Now: A new three-year strategy for people with learning disabilities* (DH, 2009). This document offers a future vision for the health and care of individuals with learning disabilities and their families and the policy objectives include many of the values explored above by the nurses who were interviewed.

What is children's nursing?

Introduction

This field of practice involves working with children of all ages who are suffering from many conditions. Children's nurses deal with a range of situations, including babies born with heart complications, teenagers who have sustained broken limbs, and child-protection issues. Health problems can affect a child's development and it's vital to work with the child's family or carers to ensure that he or she does not suffer additionally from the stress of being ill or in hospital.

Children's nursing takes place in hospitals, day care centres, children's health clinics and in children's homes. As in other fields of nursing practice, care is becoming more community-based. You may do shift work to provide 24-hour care (**www.nhscareers.nhs.uk**).

What is nursing practice in children's nursing and what skills are needed?

The nurses interviewed for this discussion have worked in general hospitals and also identified children's hospitals and specialised units, such as intensive care or accident and emergency departments. They also have experience of working in community practice. Read about their experiences of what children's nurses do in CN Excerpt 1.

CN Excerpt 1

Interviewer: What is nursing practice in children's nursing?

There's all sorts of situations depending on what ward you work on, what area you work in, whether you work within the community, where you would look after well children, or whether you work on an acute ward where you would look after . . . some maybe well children but extremely poorly children . . . at the ICU [intensive care unit].

I think that the main part within children's services specifically is working, in whatever situation you're working in, is working in partnership with people. It's about planning care for children along with the families and medics as well. And I think that's the same in children's services, whatever situation you're in, be it at home or in hospital.

Absolutely, definitely, and I think that the thing of negotiating the care, and I know it's really clichéd, but that's really important that you communicate and negotiate the care with the parents and the children, if they're old enough.

I guess it is taking sort of specific scenarios on a day-to-day basis, it involves the basic things like carrying out observations, temperatures, blood pressures . . . you might carry out more specialist observations in some areas, giving medicines that are prescribed.

. . . but also playing with the children, talking to the children, talking to parents . . .

Maintaining their safety.

I think if you're just looking at the community element, you're still doing a lot of observations but it's slightly different isn't it? You might be monitoring things like heights and weights and things like that, and also looking at the same kinds of observations in the community for the sick child if you're working as a children's community nurse, so these kinds of things are going on as well.

There's a big element of monitoring and health promotion, I think, as well, isn't there, and providing information and advice.

Activity 7.5	*Reflection*

After reading this excerpt, try to think about children's nursing.

- How was children's nursing defined and what features were identified as important?
- Jot down the most important points about children's nursing that you read and reflect on these.
- Was the way the nurses described their practice something that you expected or did it surprise you at all?

Brief outline answers are given at the end of the chapter.

The nurses identified that their work included many clinical skills, including monitoring and assessment in order to plan and provide care. Of course, they only offered some simple examples of these practical and clinical skills, but they do offer an idea of what children's nurses do. To find out more about the clinical skills of children's nursing, take a look at Kelsey and McEwing (2008) or Hockenbury and Wilson (2007).

Activity 7.6	*Communication*

Communication was identified as important for children's nurses, and it is referred to throughout this book as a key element of nursing.

After reading through CN Excerpt 1:

- Jot down your ideas about the aspects of communication that are particularly important for children's nursing.
- Do you think communication skills may be different for children's nurses when compared to other areas of nursing?
- Use the following text to support your learning:

Crawford, P and Brown, B (2009) Communication, in Mallik, M, Hall, C and Howard, D (eds) *Nursing Knowledge and Practice: A decision making approach*, 3rd edition, Edinburgh: Elsevier.

Outline answers are given at the end of the chapter.

Now read CN Excerpt 2 about the skills needed by children's nurses. Here, the nurses discuss their work using communication in greater depth. Reflect on whether you identified the same aspects in your practical activity and reading as they have done.

CN Excerpt 2

Interviewer: What are the skills needed in children's nursing?

Good communication, to be able to communicate well is a vital skill.

Also to be versatile, I guess, with what we just said about all the accessibility and the differences in the job you've got to be versatile and transfer your skills from one area to another . . .

. . . And from one age to another. You've got to be just as able to understand the parameters of taking temperature or a pulse or blood pressure on a baby as you are on a 17-year-old. And also understand in terms of communicating that difference in ages, you've got to be very flexible in that.

I think you almost have to be a jack-of-all-trades in terms of children because you're subjected to a huge range of, like you say, ages, but also the normal differences between families. And you really have to be able to adapt your communication, not just to different developmental ages but different families, different intellectual levels in parenting. Because communication's such a big thing in children's nursing, I think that's really important.

I think for any parent in hospital overnight [it is important] to take part, and the role of the nurse is sort of to empower them to still be able to do the normal things for their child that they might do at home. Like clean teeth . . .

. . . That takes a lot of confidence, because in a way you are making, you're being able to say 'I can do this, and I can also give it back to you' and I think that does differentiate children's nursing from a lot of other nursing in that a lot of what children's nurses do is have that knowledge and choose when to use it, and choose when to say 'and I'm going to help you and support you in this, do you need any further help or are you quite happy to do it for yourself?' Keeping the family and empowering the family is quite important.

But it's definitely important to have, like you said, the balance of actually being astute enough to realise when the parents maybe do need help and aren't left to do everything, because that can be a risk of getting this recognition. And parents are there so much, and they do so much of the care that we need to be aware that sometimes the parents will need help and know when to give that help.

And sometimes they need a break too.

In the above excerpt, the nurses discussed their skills in communication, but they also talked about their role in enabling and empowering parents to take on the care of their children in an appropriate way. This is quite difficult for new children's nurses and nursing students sometimes, because they have to know how to perform many aspects of nursing care, but then they may not be the people who are actually giving this care directly to their patients. They need to ensure that parents feel involved to a point where they are able, but that, if needed, the nurse can step in. For student nurses this presents unique challenges, as they may sometimes feel as though they have limited opportunities to learn skills in the clinical setting because parents may be giving care to their children. In actual fact, they need to be more skilled in these practices in order to be able not only to perform skills to a high level, but also to teach parents and children and then appropriately assess capacity for their involvement.

In schools of nursing, these issues are recognised for children's nursing students and many different mechanisms are put in place to ensure that nurses do become skilled practitioners by the time that they become registered. These include the use of simulation equipment, where skills are practised on life-sized dummies within skill laboratories, as well as focused skills opportunities and assessments identified within real practice settings. However, if you do feel frustrated or challenged about the experiences you feel you can get while in your practice placements, it is important that you talk with your personal tutor and your practice mentor, as they can help you.

Although there are some challenges associated with children's nursing, such as the one described above, there are many parts of the work that are immensely satisfying. In CN Excerpts 3 and 4, the nurses talk more about the best parts and the particular challenges they have found during their careers.

CN Excerpt 3

Interviewer: What are the best parts of the job in children's nursing?

I think the children, the children and the parents are the best thing about being a children's nurse. The relationship that you . . . even for kids who aren't in our ward for a long time, but to actually know that you've done a good job, and you do get that feedback from parents, and you do get that feedback from kids, and that – for me – is always the best thing. The actual knowing, really trying to do your best and really trying to make a difference, and it sounds a bit clichéd, but it's true. Really trying to make a difference to needy kids, and parents. And if you actually get positive feedback from parents, I think that is always really great.

I think that's the same in the community [setting] as well. I think if you're working within a health centre or you're working within a children's centre and you're working with children and families, the sense that the child has just communicated something that you may have been doing an assessment or whatever with that child and family and they've had a good experience, and you feel you've got a good relationship, and you feel that you've been able to achieve what you wanted, but they've come out of it achieving, you know, you've achieved what they want as well. And that's really quite important.

I think working in the settings that I've done, working with a lot of children with long-term patients, or in hospital for a long period of time. I think I've always felt the best thing is to be allowed into such a privileged position in people's families. Not just the child and the parents, but their extended families . . . And I think that's one of the best parts for me.

The nurses identified that their job satisfaction was highly related to the relationships they build, and the outcomes that they achieve with the children and their families during their work. Interestingly, although they suggested that this was the best part of the job, they also found that managing these relationships also presented many challenges for them. In CN Excerpt 4, read about how they recognise and cope with these.

CN Excerpt 4

Interviewer: What are the challenges of being a children's nurse?

One of the main challenges is that it can be a very stressful job; you feel you're trying to split yourself in too many directions, between too many people. And I think, again, this is probably speaking personally, not giving too much of yourself can be a bit of a challenge as well, in not getting too emotionally involved. I think that's really easy to do.

Yes, it's not the kind of job you turn off at the end of the day very easily at all, is it? And really, when you're talking about other people's lives, should it be? But at the same time you have to manage that in order to have a life of your own.

Maintaining a professional balance – confidentiality versus acting in the best interest of the patient

What is most important in this discussion is the complexity of managing emotional relationships with patients and striking a balance in maintaining a professional relationship and being caring individuals. In nursing, you must maintain caring relationships with your patients and their families at all times, but these have to be professional. This may seem really obvious, but in practice it is sometimes difficult for new nurses. For teenagers and young people this can be particularly difficult, as teenage patients do see younger nurses as peers and people in whom they can confide. This has advantages and disadvantages. There are issues about what the patients may say to you, and how much you can keep in confidence, if they say they do not want you to tell anyone, and there is a potential risk of unprofessional relationships and subsequently unrealistic expectations developing in either patients or nurses. Recognising these situations, and seeking support and advice from mentors very quickly, is important.

While you have to maintain professional relationships with the child and family and not allow any relationship to develop inappropriately, student nurses in the children's field also worry that this might mean that they should not show the emotions they are feeling. Again, this is a question of balance, as showing no emotion when a child dies or a family receives very bad news may feel very wrong and, certainly, there is a need to show compassion, which in itself is emotive.

Research summary

Turner and Thomas (2006) offer a guide for talking with children and young people about death and dying, while Thompson and Hall (2007) explore the concerns of student nurses surrounding death and dying in children. Finally, Crawford and Way (2009) consider the legal and ethical dilemmas faced by children's nurses in respect of withdrawal of treatment for children.

Finally, the nurses consider the challenges associated with not being prejudicial in the care that they give. Difficult situations such as those described by the children's nurses in CN Excerpt 5 arise in all areas of nursing and can be challenging for nurses.

CN Excerpt 5

Interviewer: Are there any more challenges you can think of?

You've got to put your prejudices aside in children's. I think you do in other areas as well, you know, in the emergency department if you're looking after people who come in, teenagers who come in and have had a scrap and they come in injured. You don't want to ask what they did to the other person or anything like it. But you know you kind of want to know that, but really in a way it's not for you to be able to make a judgement about whether it was the right thing that they hit that other child or, you know, it's quite complicated really.

We had quite a few cases where, when I worked in the city, where children were brought in having had hands and feet broken because they'd done various things they shouldn't have done. And people did make judgements and that, it was wrong, at the end of the day you still had a young person who was in there with broken hands, broken feet, who needed to be care for, who needed pain relief. Regardless of whether they'd been right or wrong . . .

. . . No, and I think you can extend that as well to children who take overdoses, children who come in drunk. There are so many challenges for young people and you've got to be very cautious in the management of those in a way that is absolutely non-judgemental really, whatever your perceptions you've kind of got to put them a bit aside.

It's not our role to judge them, in order to care for them . . .

And that's quite hard I think . . .

It can be, especially if they're difficult as well, or aggressive, or their behaviour's challenging.

The nurses in the above excerpt discussed major issues and highlighted different concerns relating to their care of young people. There is a very wide role for children's nurses, from the care of tiny babies, through to the management of teenagers and their families. Sometimes children of different ages are cared for in areas specific for their age and so it is possible to choose a career option that is age-related. This includes working in the neonatal unit, or in a specialised adolescent care unit. At other times, the work of the children's nurse may cross a wide range of ages, for example in a children's ward or in a health centre.

Activity 7.7   *Reflection*

It is very useful to reflect sometimes on where you would like to be in five years' time. This gives the opportunity for you to have a vision or a measuring stick, which, while flexible, can be used to reconsider your future options. Try to imagine where you would like to be and then think of the possible stepping stones towards achieving your goal.

As this activity is based on your own reflection, there is no outline answer at the end of the chapter.

As well as identifying the types of work that children's nurses could do, the nurses also discussed how you might get a job, recognising that you need to apply to the place of employment where you wish to work. They also identified that jobs were not always available and you may not get your first choice of work to begin with. In children's nursing, as in many other areas of nursing in the UK, there is localised fluctuation in employment opportunity, although nationally there has been a persistent shortage of children's nurses over the last 30 years. The demographic forecast relating to the workforce in healthcare in the UK does not suggest that this will change for the better (Buchan and Aiken, 2008). This is good news for new nurses, but a headache for employers. However, it does not mean that you can just walk into a job. Employers have increased the rigour of their employment processes in recent years in response to Government targets for safer healthcare environments. In children's nursing particularly, but also in some other areas, employers are testing potential candidates for maths and basic skills ability as well as conducting interviews. It is important to find out as much as you can about the employers when you are looking for a job, and prepare yourself well.

Finally, in CN Excerpt 6, the children's nurses were asked about their vision for the future of children's nursing. They talk about whether children should be looked after by people with specific training in caring for children and their families, which has been a subject of debate in the media. See if you agree with their views.

CN Excerpt 6

Interviewer: What is your vision of nursing in the children's nursing field of practice in the future?

I think it'll become more community-based, won't it? There'll be less jobs in the acute Trusts, and I think that certainly in the time that I've been practising you can already see the evidence that children in hospital are sicker and need more complex care. And so,

continued opposite . . .

continued . . .

therefore, that must mean that the children in the community are having more complex care. And so, in future, I think that's going to increase, in terms of there's going to be sicker children being looked after at home, so less in hospital.

Conclusion

This section presented the nature of children's nursing as it is seen by those participating in it in a range of different careers. It shows that there are many elements observed in other fields of nursing that are applied in a unique way in relation to the care of children. There are also specific elements that cannot be applied in their areas, which makes the nursing of children uniquely different. In England, as well as being subject to nursing drivers, including the *Essence of Care* benchmarks and the Children's NSF (DH, 2004d), children's nurses are also a part of an integrated service with a legal commitment to working within the Children Act (HM Government, 2004) and the Every Child Matters (ECM) agenda (DCSF, 2003).

Concept summary: What is Every Child Matters?

Every Child Matters is a governmental initiative. The Government's aim is for every child, whatever their background or circumstances, to have the support they need to:

- be healthy;
- stay safe;
- enjoy and achieve;
- make a positive contribution;
- achieve economic well-being.

For further details, go to **www.everychildmatters.gov.uk/aims**

What is mental health nursing?

Introduction

Mental health nurses work with children, adults and older people with various types of mental health needs. As a registered mental health nurse you may work with clients in their own homes, in residential units, in the NHS or in private specialist hospital services and secure units. The work involves helping people to recover from their problems or come to terms with them in order to maximise their life potential. Mental health nurses liaise with psychiatrists, occupational therapists, GPs, social workers and other health professionals to plan and deliver care using a multidisciplinary client-centred approach (Riddick, 2010).

What is nursing practice in the field, and what skills are needed?

For mental health nursing, the emphasis for caring is strongly based on the focus of developing, maintaining and ending therapeutic human relationships. The work undertaken by mental health nurses in the UK today is wide-ranging and offers many exciting opportunities for individuals entering this profession. The nurses talking in these excerpts have worked in a range of nursing areas within mental healthcare, including acute and community settings, and in educating new mental health nurses within a university, and the views of recently qualified and more experienced nurses are included. MH Excerpt 1 collects points from the nurses' talk about the nature of mental health nursing as they see it, and the underpinning values they see as important for a mental health nurse today. Later, they focus on a case study described by one of the group, which identified the situation of a client in the community who had developed a difficult relationship with his family and neighbours as the result of appearing different from them. In the excerpt, the nurses consider values, but also perceptions of mental health nursing, tackling issues such as fear and anxieties that are commonly identifiable in society in relation to mental healthcare. Read about their views and what being a mental health nurse means to them.

MH Excerpt 1

Interviewer: What is nursing practice in the field of mental health?

. . . for me, it's about human skills more than anything else. Being a good listener, a good communicator, and I think, alongside that, understanding obviously there's a kind of intellectual understanding. But I would observe the need for the human skills of compassion to go alongside that understanding.

. . . and I suppose underpinning that there are certain values that are needed for mental health nursing. And some of those values about human rights and justice, social justice and things like that . . . that I would say inform and should inform mental health nurse practice.

I think a lot of people, when they think about people with mental health problems, they're generally quite scared often, a bit fearful of maybe those people being a bit violent towards them and that actually a lot of these things are stereotypes and it's often that people have had really difficult life experiences, and their sort of mental and psychological and emotional distress makes sense in the context of those life experiences that you were talking about. You know, you were talking about the guy being scared of his neighbours, but yet he'd had a really good relationship with his neighbours and they'd rejected him, and, you know, that say, some of his . . . what . . . in . . . some of his, kind of, unusual beliefs, what some people call delusions, actually make sense in terms of his past experiences.

Mental health nursing leads to understanding, the level of understanding that, if somebody is behaving in a certain kind of way, it's so easy to just categorise, and pigeonhole, and stereotype: 'this person's mad', 'this person's ill', or whatever. What we

continued opposite . . .

continued . . .

need to be doing is to be understanding the bigger picture, like you've done, with the person's history and social situation, relationships, circumstances, and people don't live in vacuums. People are social beings in a social world, and there are invariably some kinds of social or relational difficulties that often impact upon the person's psychological well-being. And I think that's what mental health nurses need to do, critically, is to understand the person in the context of society, relationships. And that's why mental health nursing is primarily relational, because human beings are relational and problems exist in a relational context.

. . . Perhaps one of the other things that we should acknowledge is that we agree on the importance of the social aspects and the focus on understanding people in terms of their society and their context. But there are a whole other range of bodies of thought that would disagree with us, that perhaps would focus on the more medicalised understanding of mental distress in that it is caused by chemical imbalances in someone's brain that affects their behaviour. And I think really that's something again to identify as a challenge in that we don't have any concrete answers in terms of mental health.

Activity 7.8   *Reflection*

Think about your life . . . what has influenced you to become the person you are today? Jot down your ideas into a concept map.

Look at the map you've drawn. It is likely you've had lots of ideas, and the list is never really exhaustive, but things you might have included could be:

*   your family and relationships and your experiences of these;
*   your health and that of your family and friends;
*   how you have been treated as a person by others;
*   how old you are;
*   your cultural beliefs and values and those of others;
*   where you live;
*   how much money you have;
*   where you went to school;
*   your friends;
*   which country you live in and which area;
*   whether you are from a rural or urban community, a wealthy or poor one;
*   whether there has been conflict in your life, or distress;
*   whether you have ever moved countries.

Now look again at the items you've included – think of how your life might be different if some of these aspects were removed or were never there. What might cause you the greatest happiness or distress?

continued overleaf . . .

continued . . . •••

Refer back to the excerpt above and try to reflect on how others see you. Think about what the nurses have said about the relational elements of mental health nursing, understanding how individuals become in need of care and the need to contextualise those needs within the social and relational contexts of people's lives.

As this activity is based on your own life and reflection, there is no outline answer at the end of the chapter.

What skills do mental health nurses need?

In order to manage mental health nursing, many skills are needed. In the second excerpt the nurses talk about some of the skills of mental health nursing, what they are and how they can be used to support the people who need their care. To illustrate this further, MH Excerpt 2 is followed by two case studies described by the nurses interviewed. Each case study is prefaced by a short introduction setting the context of the situation.

MH Excerpt 2

Interviewer: What skills do mental health nurses need?

I suppose in terms of skills and clinical skills, if you're thinking about nurse training, it is a bit different [in other fields of practice] because these don't tend to be so practically based, but more technologically based, but there are certain skills or certain interventions or certain strategies that you can learn about that help you in working with certain people. So that might be about relaxation techniques, in learning how to help people relax, or it might be about managing anxiety and different ways of challenging feelings of anxiety, and the same with voices maybe, helping people learn about different strategies that help them cope with voices. And that's kind of some of the skills or ways of working with people, your kind of practical things, that a nurse might find themselves doing.

Creative approaches, getting people to do some drama, and drawing, and painting, and singing and playing music . . .

I view it as enabling people to build a toolkit of things that will help them maintain a lifestyle that is satisfactory to them. So whatever their goal is, what will they need to do to reach that goal? And what skills will they need to hold to be able to do that?

Applying skills of mental health nursing in practice

In the following case study, the nurse talks about the application of skills to help the nurse support a client in managing voices that he heard, so that he could return to college.

Case study

'One example of a chap that I used to work with, who was a really intelligent chap, but heard quite derogatory voices, and would shout out loud to them to tell them to shut up. But wanted to go back to college to do his GCSEs and that involved a lot of work in terms of coping skills, managing his anger and responding to his voices, to be able to sit within a classroom and concentrate for an hour and have his learning to achieve. And it took us probably two and a half years to even get to the classroom situation, including taxi journeys there where we didn't quite make it and things like that. It took quite a long time, and a few frightened taxi drivers along the way as well! But, yeah, in that situation it was really about equipping this chap, or helping to equip himself, with those skills and they would be different for whatever situation or whatever person . . . .'

The next case study returns to the man discussed earlier in MH Excerpt 1, who had relational difficulties with his family and neighbours. In the case study, the nurse talks about using skills to build a therapeutic relationship and support the man's care needs.

Case study

'. . . when I picked this chap up, he'd spent all these years quite isolated in his home, becoming very frightened, angry, towards his mum and towards his neighbours, and [would] go out and have outbursts in the street. You know, "stop watching me", and all this kind of thing. So it turned into what people would see as, like, stereotypical "mad" way of acting. When I started to work with him and we went back and looked at his history, and his past, and who he'd been and his identity and his roles, that had felt like it was completely eroded. That all that was left of him now, all that he saw of himself, was a burden really, and a mad person in society. And because of that he had no worth to society and no belief in what he could offer. And that was our starting point really, because, really identifying what, well, first of all gaining this chap's trust, because he hadn't really worked with anyone over a long period of time.

He would start to believe that they were involved in these kinds of plots against him, and feeding information to the neighbours. So starting off with that and looking at what were this guy's ambitions, what was he as a person. And really trying to convince him that he had more to offer. And I suppose that was very much informed by a strength perspective, looking at what he had achieved in his past and what would enable him to achieve those things, and what did he want for his future.

I felt my role in that was a lot about me having belief in his ability, and where he didn't see it . . . To reassure him, I suppose, and reiterate what he had to offer, and the meaning that he could rebuild in his life. And we took very small steps, and the first one was about having driving lessons again, he did have the licence but hadn't driven for years and years and so he started with driving lessons, and that opened up a huge world for him, so he had independence and he would hire a car for a weekend and go out on long drives to country pubs that he had been to in his past. And we built it up from there really and built up on small successes, and I view him really and somebody that, kind of, I don't know what the word is, as an example of how a relationship and a belief in somebody's abilities can make a real difference to their lives, and I think that's how I view my role as a mental health carer.'

What are the best parts of working as a mental health nurse and what challenges are there?

MH Excerpt 3

Interviewer: So, what's the best thing about being a mental health nurse?

I think it's always, mental health nursing always provides, every day provides fresh challenges.

You never have the same day twice . . .

No. and I never, ever, dreaded going to work. Mental health nursing has been enjoyable for me.

And there's something about this enormous privilege of working with some of the most vulnerable people in society. But also about this enormous privilege of working in an area of people's lives that's normally closed. You know, people open up to you. That you're invited into very private areas of people's . . . [lives], it's a great privilege.

I think that working in some of the areas where we've all worked, that is a huge challenge – because people have been let down by relationships over and over again throughout their lives, it has been reinforced to them. So when you did get to that stage, where people were able to be open and honest with you, that felt like a huge reward . . . that you could really make a difference.

What are the practicalities – what kinds of different work can mental health nurses do?

This section uses the excerpt to identify and discuss the type of work that mental health nurses might undertake in their practice.

Activity 7.9   *Decision making*

Before you read the next section, jot down on a piece of paper all the roles and jobs that you can imagine mental health nurses working in today. If you go to practice placements in mental health settings, you could see whether you could add to your list, and also you can add ideas from your reading. Try also to expand on some of these roles.

- What is the nature of the work and what would a career in that area of mental health look like?
- How do these people work with others in the multiprofessional healthcare team?

continued opposite . . .

---

continued . . . ●●

This work can be placed in your portfolio, and will help you to meet competency outcomes relating to care management and to personal and professional development. Now read MH Excerpt 4 and see if you identified as many kinds of work as the nurses did!

As this activity is based on your own reflection and observations, there is no outline answer at the end of the chapter.

MH Excerpt 4

Interviewer: What kinds of different work can mental health nurses do?

Drug and alcohol services, because one thing that really, really complicates mental health nursing is, we are often working with some of the most damaged people in society that often turn to substance misuse. You know, you can get children as young as 7 drug taking, and heroin addicts by 14 and things like that. And people get caught up in the criminal justice system. And with the closure of the asylums, people that may have been in an asylum actually end up in prison.

That's another area where mental health nurses can work, isn't it? It's in-reach teams that go into prison to offer support to the populations.

So there is that whole area of mental health nursing, that works in that difficult, complex area of people with drug problems, alcohol problems, forensic history, both in-patient and the community.

We've spoken quite a lot about people who've had mental health problems for a long time and at times are quite damaged. But obviously mental health nursing can be about a lot more than that and there is, you know, we know statistics of one in four people experiencing mental health problems and 90 per cent of those kind of initial contacts being in GP surgeries. So I think working with people in mental distress in primary care is a huge kind of area which is really starting to take off.

Most GP surgeries have a mental health nurse in them, which GPs can refer people to, to see for a short time, often to deal with things like bereavement and that kind of thing.

. . . and there are teams that support people in accident and emergency as well, for people who might have self-harmed and mental health nurses go in and do assessments and offer short-term support . . .

. . . liaison

. . . there's loads of services for older people with mental health problems, either that have had mental health problems for their lives, diagnosed with schizophrenia and have gone into old age with problems, physical problems, as well as the mental health problems. But also, of course, dementia and Alzheimer's.

continued overleaf . . .

continued . . .

... And again some really interesting, creative ways with working with people in those settings. Things like 'validation' ... Life story work and getting friends and family to bring in photos of the person and create the story of their life, and working with the person around that.

We ought to include acute in-patient care in our discussion, where nurses would find themselves working shifts in a hospital ward, it's all very medically orientated.

Something we haven't mentioned is the sort of post-traumatic stress work that mental health nurses can do. And it is emerging as an increasingly important area and certainly locally there's a mental health nurse, he is a mental health nurse, isn't he? Who works internationally in sort of crisis zones, you know, earthquake and disaster areas to offer psychological support so that would be another career pathway I suppose ... and travel opportunities.

What about the practicalities? Getting a job and career opportunities in mental health nursing

Activity 7.10	*Reflection*

In MH Excerpt 5, the nurses talk about the practicalities of getting jobs and of some of the career opportunities available for mental health nurses today.

Before you read, try to imagine where you would like your career in mental health to take you. Use the activity above to think about the kinds of jobs available to you and then try to imagine what you would like to be doing in five years' time.

Note this information for inclusion in your portfolio. Put it where you can review it in a year's time to see if your ideas have changed.

As this activity is based on your own reflection, there is no outline answer at the end of the chapter.

MH Excerpt 5

Interviewer: What career opportunities are available on qualification?

[There is] ... the opportunity to work quite autonomously because so much of the work has been based in the community. That automatically means that mental health nurses have the opportunity to move up the grades ... and there's greater flexibility in that. It doesn't work in all circumstances, but you know, I think going back a few years even in mental

continued opposite . . .

continued . . .

health, you used . . . you had to have two years with in-patients before you could work in the community. You had to be an E grade before you could become an F grade or whatever. I think that those kinds of barriers are disappearing really, and if you can show that you've got the relevant experience then most of the opportunities are open to you.

. . . and there is no kind of speciality. I think it's OK to move across specialisms . . .

Not every area has this, but certainly my own experience I think every job I've gone for I've been interviewed by a service user, a service user and carer panel.

Normally, I mean, there have been a few hiccups in the last couple of years, but normally there are jobs for people to get into . . .

I actively chose my first job in an area that I was interested in working in and I'd got experience working, I felt confident to go there. It was a nice position to be in for a newly qualified nurse. But I think with limited positions available people might be forced to take positions that do not suit their philosophy, it might not suit their way of working. And that's perhaps a problem that might affect attrition rates and others' experiences.

If you work in acute for six months, it doesn't mean that you need to kind of stay there. It means that you could get and maybe get a job in drugs and alcohol or . . .

It's all good experience no matter what. Yeah.

Not all jobs involve shift work . . .

No, the majority don't really now with the focus more on community.

But perhaps that is something that in the future is becoming more flexible, isn't it? Not being so rigid, and traditionally community teams work 9–5 Monday to Friday and that's that, and in response to service users' needs and the development of services that's changing.

The nurses talk a lot about the influence of the service user in mental health, both in terms of the type of care they need to give and in relation to the way that those who use mental health services influence the service and can help to assist practitioners in developing a service that is responsive. This may mean that new job candidates are interviewed by a panel including mental health service users in some areas.

Activity 7.11   *Reflection and research*

Try to think about the mental health services that have been described above. If you were in need of help from these services:

- What would you like to see?
- What would you be asking candidates about in a job interview if they were going to be caring for you?

continued overleaf . . .

continued . . . ●●●

Use your own experiences of any healthcare you or your family may have needed – try to reflect on what was important for you.

Thinking about these elements from the perspective of a service can help you to be responsive as a practitioner and sensitive to some of the needs of others. Support this reflection through reading about some service-user experiences of services found on the Perceptions Forum website (**www.voicesforum.org.uk/nvf.htm**). There is also a useful resource to extend your knowledge around mental health issues managed by the Mental Health Alliance (**www.mentalhealthalliance.org.uk**).

As this activity is based on your own reflection, there is no outline answer at the end of the chapter.

A vision for the future of mental health nursing

Finally, the nurses were asked to consider their future vision for mental health nursing. Read MH Excerpt 6 and see if you agree with them. What vision would you have for excellence in mental health nursing in the future?

MH Excerpt 6

Interviewer: Do you have a vision for the future of nursing in mental health?

. . . Less dependency on the drug companies, less dependency on prescriptions. Yes, some people need some drugs some of the time; that doesn't mean that all the people that come into our service need all the drugs all the time. And it's that whole concept of hope, if we can help to develop a mental health field of the future that inspires hope in, amongst nurses in their practice, and subsequently amongst our clients, our patients, whoever they are of the future. It's about healing in society, it's about adjusting social injustice and social ills, and if mental health nursing can contribute to that healing of society, then for me that is a vision that I want to pursue. So it's all very uplifting.

It is, in the way that hope can be quite infectious, can't it? If you believe in somebody for long enough, then they will believe in themselves and the same . . .

. . . and I think society has moved forwards, you know, we are moving forwards . . . and I think mental health field needs to continue to have the optimism that society is . . . improving, and mental health nursing is part of that improvement in how we treat the most vulnerable people in society.

. . . and perhaps that's the key isn't it? Viewing people as the most vulnerable as opposed to the people to be frightened of. Maybe that's . . . and I think there are shifts in that opinion in the way that mental health problems are being reported in the media has been shown to be changed, and all that will help along that journey.

continued opposite . . .

continued . . .

. . . for me, I think that the missing link is law to prohibit discrimination on the grounds of mental health, and law that will defend people's rights not to be stigmatised . . .

Yeah, in the way they have for racial equality, gender equality, physical disability, yeah.

What is adult nursing?

Introduction

Adult nurses provide medical care to, and support the recovery of, patients suffering from acute and long-term illnesses – diseases such as diabetes or arthritis, or problems requiring surgery. They focus on the needs of the patient rather than the illness or condition. They also promote good health and well-being through education. Nurses plan and carry out care within a multi-disciplinary team, but are the main point of contact for patients.

Adult nurses work mainly in hospitals, although they are playing an increasingly prominent role in the community, attached to a health centre or general practice and in residential homes, specialist units, schools and hospices (Clark, 2009).

What is nursing practice in adult healthcare and what skills are needed?

In AN Excerpt 1 from an interview with a group of experienced nurses from the adult field of practice, the participants talk about the most important parts of being qualified to nurse adults, and also some skills that they need in their work. As you read their discussion, see if you can identify what these are. Remember, these are examples and do not cover everything, but they do offer you a flavour.

AN Excerpt 1

Interviewer: Right. So, what does a nurse in the field of adult healthcare do?

Well, you're expecting nurses to be assessing and evaluating patients in their care. Delivering care.

Working as part of a team . . .

Communicating with the patients and relatives . . .

Being aware of when things are going wrong with patients and highlighting it to the right person.

continued overleaf . . .

continued . . . •••

Caring about people as well . . . because I think sometimes the caring element can be forgotten, can't it?

. . . And it's not just about that person, it's about their family, and their friends, and the people around. Because I bet you spend hours with the relatives, and friends . . .

I think it's also acting as support for junior members of staff. So whether that's the students that are just coming up along behind, or auxiliary staff, or domestic staff, or, you know, anyone that's in a more junior position. They'll need supporting as well, which can happen quite quickly on qualifying, but then you sort of expect it to really.

. . . and a lot of physical care and physical conditions as well, isn't it? You've got to have quite a breadth of knowledge even within a specialty to be able to cope with everything that comes your way. And prescribing, you're doing prescribing at the moment aren't you?

I think the skills needed to be an adult nurse for me, I think, what you said [X], the most important thing is the caring. It is for me, it's always been about, you know, like gut instinct of why you ever wanted to be a nurse in the first place. And yes, you've got to have all the professional, you know, educational skills and all that side that goes with it. But actually, why you're in nursing in the first place is really important. You know, I think, you can lose sight of that.

And I think you've got to be adaptable. Particularly in this day and age.

Problem-solving skills as well are essential. We've got to be good problem solvers haven't we?

Think on your feet . . .

Stop doing one thing to start doing another and go back. And that's kind of the norm to do in adult nursing really. To be thrown out of one situation and do something that's a priority.

. . . And you've got to keep up to date with such a lot of stuff as well. You know, so you've got to be a lifelong learner . . .

Activity 7.12   *Reflection*

After reading this excerpt, try to think about adult nursing.

*   How was adult nursing defined and what features were identified as important?
*   Was the way the nurses described their practice something that you expected or did it surprise you at all?
*   What skills did you see in the nurses' discussion that are important to an adult nurse?

Brief outline answers are given at the end of the chapter.

It is no surprise that, when nursing literature is explored, many of these skills are taught and assessed during preparation to be come a qualified nurse, but it is important to see how these nurses are using their skills in their work. The skills outlined by the adult nurses have focused on quite broad knowledge and practice that is transferable to many settings. These skills complement many specific nursing skills relating to observation and monitoring, and to clinical practices for caring and treating patients. I am sure you can think of many examples, but to start you off, think about washing and bathing, maintaining hygiene, managing infection control and maintaining dignity, as well as skills in administering medicines, changing dressings and managing catheters, infusion tubes and drains when patients are very sick. A useful text for reference in considering these fundamental skills and procedures is Dougherty and Lister (2007).

Once qualified, you are at the beginning of a long career that may change in focus within the field of practice you have chosen. You may decide to specialise in a specific field of practice. In AN Excerpt 2, a nurse who has specialised in adult respiratory care talks about how her work complements that of others in the multidisciplinary team. Notice how she describes the importance of being able to assess all her patients' needs and then refer them to others for care to be given.

AN Excerpt 2

Interviewer: What other aspects do you think are important?

I think that is one of the things, obviously, I see when I go out in the community, because I go out as a respiratory nurse; if I go and see a patient who has developed a pressure sore, you have to get somebody else to come in and look at the pressure sore.

But [sigh], you know, your gut instinct is to treat your patients holistically, so you look at all those situations and do as much as you can do; obviously when you're working in a different environment you have to work to the different rules and regulations, if you like, of that area, whether it's secondary care, primary care, whatever . . . But it doesn't stop you doing the assessment bit. That's the important thing, isn't it? You know, I've always said we don't just go in and look at that bit, you look at the whole bit, but then you refer on as appropriate, to whoever needs to do it.

So it's about knowing other people's roles, and where you sit within that team.

Activity 7.13   *Critical thinking*

Did the fact that the respiratory nurse may have to refer patients with a pressure sore surprise you? This is important, so that the respiratory nurse can focus upon her special knowledge and practice.

continued overleaf . . .

continued . . .

- Think about your own experiences in working as a team, perhaps in playing sport or in working in employment. How did you divide up the tasks to be done? Did you identify particular expertise or share the work with everyone doing the same?
- Jot down the structure of these different teams. Try critically to appraise whether the approach to team management worked in each situation.
- Recall this experience in your next nursing practice learning experience.
- Explore the teams working in the practice setting and identify who does which tasks. Is there overlap and is the method effective? How could it be improved?

As this activity is based on your own reflection, there is no outline answer at the end of the chapter.

These considerations are important when thinking about the managerial aspect of delivering effective care and healthcare. Managers increasingly have to justify their use of resources and will consider the skill mix and expertise in their teams to ensure effective practice.

Going back to the excerpt, it is important to identify that not all nurses in the community are specialists, just as not all doctors specialise within their clinical practice. It is important for the NHS to be able to offer many different types of nursing. Other clinical specialist nurses include those who specialise in managing asthma, heart disease, epilepsy, diabetes, kidney disease, tissue viability, and cancer and palliative care. All these nurses work alongside district nurses and hospital nurses to provide specialist care for patients when it is needed. These roles usually need extra study and experience in practice, but offer future expert opportunities for adult nurses after qualification.

What are the best parts of being an adult nurse and what challenges are there?

In the last excerpt, the nurse sounded sad that she could not nurse the patient's pressure sore, because she felt that she wanted to look after the patient's holistic care. Sometimes nursing is challenging and our interviewees were able to offer more challenges, too, in being an adult nurse. However, they were also keen to discuss the best bits about being adult nurses. In AN Excerpt 3, read about their consideration of what the best bit is about being an adult branch nurse and what the challenges are for them.

AN Excerpt 3

Interviewer: What's the best thing about nursing adults?

Being able to help people . . . whether you are helping to make them better or whether it's that you're helping towards a peaceful death. It's all part of nursing, it's that journey along that pathway isn't it? To me that's what's the best thing for me. You know, people say

continued opposite . . .

continued . . . .

working with chronic obstructive airways disorders, that must be really depressing, because they're all old and they all die. Well, you know, they're not – there's a lot more than just that.

I'd agree with you, it's about being able to help . . .

Make a difference . . .

I think my reason would be a bit more selfish in that I think the career of nursing, that's the best thing about it, because it opens up so many doorways. Just so, so many. Here, overseas, and all the different areas of nursing. I think that's what one of the best things about the job is.

The second nurse identified career opportunity both in the UK and abroad as one of the best parts of nursing. In a later excerpt, these opportunities were reconsidered by the group. They recognised that nursing opportunities do vary, according to the current political and financial climate, and suggested that it may not be possible to have only one job as a nurse in the same place forever. Their advice for new nurses, however, was to gain some experience, before becoming too focused on a specialty.

What are the challenges of being a nurse in the adult field of practice today?

In this part of the discussion, the adult nurses (like nurses in other fields) noted financial restrictions within the NHS as particularly influential and challenging to what they were able to do in providing patient care, and in relation to their own personal development and employment security. They specifically highlighted issues relating to the frustration of becoming more experienced and feeling that their roles in practice took them away from direct patient care, as they were increasingly responsible for many administrative activities – particularly in acute hospital care. However, two issues emerge from this: first, it was recognised that this did not always happen and that a major challenge was getting a balance to be able to spend more time with patients; but, second, it was recognised that an element of nursing does relate to the completion of administrative work in order to care for patients most effectively. As shown in previous chapters, all nurses need to assess, plan, monitor and document the care that they give, but there must also be nurse leaders and managers who have a role in ensuring that shifts are covered and that patients receive good nursing care. This includes ensuring that sufficient nurses and sufficient resources are available in an appropriate environment.

Research summary

The balance between administrative duty and spending time with patients is identified as a priority in a new NHS Institute for Innovation and Improvement (NHSIII, 2008) initiative entitled *The Productive Ward: Releasing time to care*, which, among other elements, considers how to achieve spending more time with the patient.

AN Excerpt 4 continues this discussion.

AN Excerpt 4

Interviewer: What are the challenges of being a nurse in the adult field of practice?

In a hospital environment, I think as a ward unit, you get, the buck stops here if you like. Because everything that's happened, decisions that are made higher up, they sort of devolve down and it always ends up with ward staff, doesn't it?

Absolutely . . . The priority of my day as a junior sister was, how I'm going to cover the off-duty, who's off sick, and which patients can I move to other wards. That's not what I came into nursing for. I came into nursing to do nursing, and I think certainly, the higher you go up – the more restrictions on what you can do [with patients].

. . . And yet we need to keep those experienced nurses at the bedside, because patients are more critically ill these days than they used to be, in the hospital, and in the community, because they're moved out much more quickly. And yet they're often the people that are dealing with the administrative tasks . . .

But I am at the bedside quite a lot though I think . . . [Junior Sister]

You are, you are . . .

But that might be because I need to be. Do you know what I mean?

I think it depends on which ward you're on, what management structure you've got . . .

Yeah, that's right. It depends on the individual as well, I think, because I always go to the patient first rather than go to the notes, do all my notes at the patient, with the patient, I don't sit at the end of the desk, because you know, you get so much more from the patient . . .

What about the practicalities – what kinds of work can you do as an adult nurse?

In these interviews, the discussion of nurses in the adult nursing field of practice reflects their own experiences of working in a hospital setting first, with community nursing seen as a specialty. However, they also recognise that nursing in the UK is changing and it is possible to start working as a nurse in a community setting because there are jobs now that previously did not exist.

AN Excerpt 5

Interviewer: What career opportunities are available on qualification?

. . . I would say there's lots of career opportunities, but what's really important, particularly on qualification, is getting some grounding on a general medical or surgical ward, before you can start thinking about what career opportunities are out there. I think we're very quick, because there is that emphasis on postgraduate learning and courses and all the rest of it, but actually sometimes just getting that experience for a year, 18 months, to find out where you actually want to go, because I don't think you really know that on qualifying. Sometimes you have gut instincts when you do your training, people actually enjoy surgery more than medicine. But actually then, whether it's surgical, medicine or whatever, it's which speciality within those that you enjoy. So, get the grounding first, and then think about where you want to go from there.

We've had quite a few of our adult nursing students who've gone straight into the community.

Yeah, and again, I think, if you look back to five to ten years, places like primary care, A&E, ICU, you would never have got there as a newly qualified nurse.

Activity 7.14	*Reflection*

Have a look around your practice placements and in the nursing literature or, if you have been reading through this book and doing the exercises, go back and reflect on your activities in Chapter 1.

- How many different jobs can you find that adult nurses do?
- Try to find out more about the ones that interest you.
- Jot down your preferences for working as a qualified nurse in a small part of your portfolio – what do you see yourself doing if you qualified as a nurse in the adult nursing field of practice?
- Keep these ideas safe and reflect on them once a year to see if they have changed.

As this activity is based on your own observations and reflection, there is no outline answer at the end of the chapter.

Finally, the nurses explore their visions for adult nursing in the future. Remember, these are their opinions, but they do offer insight into how they see nursing changing. Read the last excerpt and see whether you agree with them.

AN Excerpt 6

Interviewer: Do you have a vision for the future of adult nursing?

I think there are big issues in terms of nursing; there seem to me to be two fields of adult nursing developing. One is the hospital-based critical care band and the other is the more community-focused long-term conditions . . . And there doesn't seem [so] much in the middle any more. Do you know what I mean? Whereas before you would have adult patients on a ward like this, for example, and some would be quite acutely ill, and some would be convalescing but not quite ready to go home, and then they'd be fairly well before they went home. But with the whole bed situation and everything it's very, very acute, isn't it? You get very sick patients who, as soon as they start to get better, they're home.

Do you think that's because of the political agenda with all this thing with managing long-term conditions? It's all the Government and the Department of Health talk about now – it's preventing admissions, reducing bed-days, managing long-term conditions, community matrons, the whole emphasis now is on keeping people at home or getting them home early . . . You think, will there be a day where they don't come into hospital at all? You know, I think that potentially, I think if we were sat here another 10, 15 years' time, there certainly won't be hospitals as big as this around because there won't be the need for it because they'll be, you know, like the . . . big health centres that are being built that are going to be mini-hospitals in the local community.

And that's a good thing, as long as all the infrastructure is out there to look after patients . . .

[general agreement]

. . . and if you talk to patients, that's definitely what they want. Pulmonary rehabilitation for instance, they don't want to come to hospital to do pulmonary rehabilitation when they can do it a mile down the road. So, the patients definitely want care closer to home. But, like you say, they need the infrastructure and the expertise out there to provide it.

And I think another issue as well is this need to focus on, in adult nursing, there's a lot more primary and secondary prevention, primary and secondary health promotion as well. There isn't a lot is there really?

Conclusion

The adult nursing field of practice offers a wide range of opportunities, ranging from working in hospital wards with patients needing skilled clinical care involving high technology and surgical intervention to nursing out in the community. It is clear that the patients that the nurses are working with are increasingly dependent and frequently very sick, whether they are in the hospital or community setting, although those nursing adults also can have roles in promoting health and preventing ill health. Unequivocally, although the nurses recognised they had to participate in many management roles, including completing paperwork and managing budgets, they valued their patient contact highly as the most important part of their roles. Adult nurses can work abroad in the EU as well as in the UK, with automatic recognition of their registration. If they travel overseas, they may have to undertake further assessment.

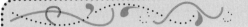

Chapter summary

This chapter has illustrated the nature of practical nursing, as it is applied to the fields of qualified nursing practice in the UK today, and has enabled you to see through the eyes of qualified nurses in the field of practice in which you are interested, which should enable you to identify experiences you may wish to explore further in your nursing course or in your work and help you to make choices about your own future career.

Throughout the chapter, the exploration of different ways of working, and the nursing needs of different patients, offers thought around the need to practise in a fair and anti-discriminatory way, acknowledging the differences in beliefs and cultural practices of individuals or groups in accordance with the NMC outcomes for proficient practice. The nurses' discussions around the team approach used in their work and the types of role undertaken should have enabled your development of knowledge and understanding around inter-professional working practices. The discussion by the nurses surrounding post-qualifying practice and learning offers an opportunity to understand more about committing to the need for CPD and personal supervision activities in order to enhance knowledge, skills, values and attitudes needed for safe and effective nursing practice, once again directly as required within the achievement of the NMC *Standards for Pre-registration Nursing Education* (2010a).

Most critically, however, this chapter has highlighted some of the real issues and concerns for nursing in the UK today and these are likely to have applicability in other countries also. This chapter has been about real nursing and about how the theory seen in the previous chapters actually works in practical situations described by the nurses themselves. It is essential to realise that core themes, such as communication, advocacy and dignity, the support for clients and their carers and families, and the privilege of being able to deliver care to another human being, are recognised within all fields of practice within nursing and are expressed powerfully within this chapter, echoing the thoughts of the authors in the first chapters of this book. What makes each field and specialty of nursing different from each other, however, is the manner in which the core themes are used and the specific needs of the clients and patients who require care. As an example, communicating with an adult is necessarily different from communicating with a child, but it is no less important in either situation, and nor is it so within mental health or learning disability care.

I hope that you have enjoyed the considerations in this chapter and that it has helped to illustrate some of the concerns for practitioners in these fields of practice. My thanks once again must go to the colleagues who have made this chapter a reality.

Activities: brief outline answers

Activity 7.1 (page 146)

It is clear that LD nursing traverses a wide range of considerations about people in our society today. Nurses must be knowledgeable about human development, the special needs of children and adults, and also issues around mental health requirements. The nurses interviewed also recognised that, with improving healthcare technology, their service is changing. Survival rates of both newborns and older people with special learning needs have increased and this means that nurses must extend their nursing knowledge around the needs of children who have very complex care requirements and adults who are entering older age.

Activity 7.3 (page 151)

An example of where the nurse's role in advocacy may be difficult or challenged relates to the situation described by the nurses where clients behaved violently. Even though the client may have been behaving wrongly, the nurse in the role of advocate would, by definition, have to advocate on their behalf. This creates a difficult balancing act, especially if others are adversely affected by violent or inappropriate behaviour. This is identified by MacDonald in her article, which also offers deeper consideration of the relationship between advocacy ethics and the nurse–patient relationship.

Activity 7.5 (page 155)

You may have concluded the following about children's nursing.

- Children's nursing is about caring for children and families together.
- Children's nurses have a good knowledge of child development in order to determine normal physical and cognitive parameters.
- Children's nurses work in partnership with other health professionals, including doctors, as mentioned – but also health visitors, social workers, physiotherapists, playworkers, teachers, occupational therapists and physiotherapists, and many more.
- Children's nurses can work with children who are well, offering advice and health promotion to families and monitoring, with children with long-term illness and with children who are sick. Some nurses work with children who are very sick. This can be in specialised units, such as intensive care, but it may be at home or in hospices, where such care can be provided.
- Children's nurses need to know how to communicate effectively as this is a large part of their role.
- Children's nurses need to play with children who are their patients and with their siblings, as part of the care they give.

Activity 7.6 (page 155)

You may have concluded some of the following.

When thinking about children's nursing it is important to consider the developmental stage of the individual and what they will be able to understand and remember reasonably. Language may need to be kept simple for young children and the time-span between communication and action should be considered. It is also critical to consider the experience of the individual. Young children may have a limited life experience and so face many new situations. While they should be included in dicussions around their care, this needs to be achieved sensitively. The principles of gaining informed consent are equally important in children's nursing, but there should be a consideration around the child's capacity to consent and also around their need for appropriate information. It may be necessary to consider using other mediums, apart from verbal communication, to get your message across (photo books, stories, dressing up and role play are all possibilities).

Children's nurses also have to communicate with a range of parents, who also have communication needs that must be assessed in order to ensure effective care. Children's nurses must work with parents to give care and the frequency and expected nature of this partnership type of arrangement with families defines children's nursing.

When working with children, skilled communicating is critical, and nurses need to be particularly skilled at developing relationships with children and building trust. This is not always easy and requires considerable skill, especially when children are frightened by events or nervous around adults outside the family circle. Hospital or healthcare admission is a particularly daunting experience for many children.

Activity 7.12 (page 172)

You may have concluded the following.

* 'Caring' is an important feature.
* Adult nursing is about more than the patient; it is about the family and relatives too.
* Adult nurses need to have a wide range of knowledge and skills relating to adult disorders and physical problems.
* Adult nurses need to keep constantly up to date with knowledge about what is happening in their practice.
* Adult nurses need specific skills including:
  * problem solving;
  * flexibility;
  * ability to support more junior staff and students with whom they work.

Further reading

Aylott, M, Battrick, C and Glasper, EA (2009) *The Wessex Manual of Children's Practical Nursing Skills.* London: Hodder and Stoughton.

This text offers a contemporary evidence base and details practice requirements for specific clinical skills in children's nursing.

Callaghan, P, Playle, J and Cooper, L (eds) (2009) *Mental Health Nursing Skills.* Oxford: Oxford University Press.

This book considers a range of skills for mental health nursing practice and includes an excellent consideration of the essence of caring in mental health.

Dougherty, L and Lister, S (2007) *The Royal Marsden Hospital Manual of Clinical Nursing Procedures*, 7th edition. London: Royal Marsden Hospital.

Nicol, M, Bavin, C, Cronin, P and Rawlings-Anderson, K (2008) *Essential Nursing Skills.* New York: Mosby.

Both of the above books offer insight and a relevant evidence base for the learning and delivery of clinical skills by nurses.

Gates, B, Edwards, HM and Atherton, H (2007) *Learning Disabilities: Towards inclusion*, 5th edition. Edinburgh: Elsevier.

This text offers a clear consideration of the work of health professionals and others in the care of people with learning disabilities. The book also offers insights from people who have learning disabilities.

Reed, S (2011) *Successful Professional Portfolios for Nursing Students*, Exeter: Learning Matters.

This book not only provides an introduction to starting and keeping a portfolio, it looks ahead to final assessments and developnig a career beyond qualifying.

Turner, M and Thomas, B (2006) *Talking with Children and Young People about Death and Dying.* London: Jessica Kingsley.

This book addresses the practicalities of working with children and young people about their experiences of death and dying. This is a particularly complex area for children's nurses, as cognitive development influences children's capacity for understanding the concept of death.

Useful websites

www.institute.nhs.uk Includes web pages on the *Productive Ward: Releasing time to care* initiative.

www.nhscareers.nhs.uk/details Offers career summaries relating to the specialties in nursing from an NHS perspective.

www.prospects.ac.uk Offers careers advice for graduates of all kinds, but gives a helpful summary on the main roles and work undertaken by nurses working within the different field specialties.

References

ACT (2004) *Integrated Multi-agency Care Pathways for Children with Life-threatening and Life-limiting Conditions.* Available online at www.act.org.uk (accessed May 2011).

Amos, D (2001) An evaluation of staff nurse role transition, *Nursing Standard* 16(3): 36–41.

Ball, J and Pike, G (2007) *Holding On: Nurses' employment and morale in 2007.* Employment Research Ltd, commissioned by the Royal College of Nursing. London: RCN. Available online at www.employment research.co.uk (accessed 23 June 2009).

Ball, J and Pike, G (2009) *Past Imperfect, Future Tense: Nurses' employment and morale in 2009.* London: RCN (Royal College of Nursing and Employment Research).

Baly, M (1995) *Nursing and Social Change,* 3rd edition. London: Routledge.

Barton, T (2007) Student nurse practitioners – a rite of passage? The universality of Van Gennep's model of social transition. *Nurse Education in Practice* 7: 338–47.

Beauchamp, TL and Childress, JF (1994) *Principles of Biomedical Ethics,* 4th edition. New York: Oxford University Press.

Becker, MH and Maiman, LA (1975) Sociobehavioural determinants of compliance with health and medical care recommendations. *Medical Care* 13(1): 10–24.

Beecroft, PC, Santner, S, Lacy, ML, Kunzman, L and Dorey, F (2006) New graduate nurses' perceptions of mentoring: six-year programme evaluation. *Journal of Advanced Nursing* 55(6): 736–47.

Bernhauser, S (2010) Degrees will equip nurses to meet future challenges in healthcare. *Nursing Times,* 106 (21): 8.

Berry, L (2004) Is image important? *Nursing Standard,* 18(23): 14–16.

Bick, C (1999) Please help! I'm newly qualified. *Nursing Standard* 14(16): 44–7.

Bolam v. Friern Hospital Management Committee (1957) 2 A11 ER 1025.

Bradley, SF (1999) Catherine Wood: children's nursing pioneer. *Paediatric Nursing,* 11(8): 15–18.

Bridges, J (1990) Literature review on the image of the nurse and the nursing media. *Journal of Advanced Nursing,* 15(7): 850–4.

British Council (2009) *About Erasmus.* Available online at www.britishcouncil.org/erasmus-about-erasmus. htm (accessed May 2011).

Brookfield, SD (1987) *Developing Critical Thinkers: Challenging adults to explore alternative ways of thinking and acting.* San Francisco, CA: Jossey Bass.

Brown, H and Edelmann, R (2000) Project 2000: a study of expected and experienced stressors and support reported by students and qualified nurses. *Journal of Advanced Nursing* 31(4): 857–64.

Brown, J and Gobbi, M (2007) Introduction to professional studies within nursing, in Brown, J and Libberton, P (2007) *Principles of Professional Studies within Nursing,* Basingstoke: Macmillan, pp3–24.

Brown, J and Libberton, P (eds) (2007) *Principles of Professional Studies in Nursing,* Basingstoke: Palgrave Macmillan.

Buchan, J and Aiken, L (2008) Solving nursing shortages: a common priority. *Journal of Clinical Nursing,* 17(24): 3262–8.

Chan, M (2007) Message from the Director General, World Health Organization. Available online at www. who.int/world-health-day/previous/2007/activities/dg_message/en/index.html (accessed May 2011).

Chitty, KK and Black, BP (2007) *Professional Nursing*, 5th edition. Philadelphia, PA: Saunders.

Clark, A (2009) *Adult Nursing: Job description and activities*. Available online at ww2.prospects.ac.uk/p/types_of_job/adult_nurse_job_description.jsp (accessed May 2011).

Clark, T and Holmes, S (2007) Fit for practice? An exploration of the development of newly qualified nurses using focus groups. *International Journal of Nursing Studies*, 44: 1210–20.

Cormack, DFS and Reynolds, W (1992) Criteria for evaluating the clinical and practical utility of models used by nurses. *Journal of Advanced Nursing*, (17)12: 1472–8.

Cox, C (2006) Bound to care. *Nursing Standard*, 21(2): 16–18.

Crawford, P and Brown, B (2009) Communication, in Mallik, M, Hall, C and Howard, D (eds) *Nursing Knowledge and Practice: A decision making approach*, 3rd edition. Edinburgh: Elsevier.

Crawford, D and Way, C (2009) Just because we can, should we? A discussion of treatment withdrawal. *Paediatric Nursing*, 21(1): 22–5.

Crombie, IK (2007) *Pocket Guide to Critical* Appraisal 2nd edition. Oxford: Blackwell.

Cronin, G and Cronin, C (2006) Why does A&E attract newly qualified registered nurses? *Accident and Emergency Nursing*, 14: 71–7.

Cummins, A (2008) Clinical supervision: the way forward? A review of the literature. *Nurse Education in Practice*, 9(3): 215–20.

Cunningham, A (1999) Nursing stereotypes. *Nursing Standard*, 13(45): 46–7.

Danbjørg, DB and Birkelund, R (2011) The practical skills of newly qualified nurses. *Nurse Education Today*, 31(2): 168–72.

Darbyshire, P (2002) Heroines, hookers and harridans: exploring popular images and representations of nurses and nursing, in Daly, J, Speedy, S, Jackson, D and Darbyshire, P (eds) *Contexts of Nursing: An introduction*. Oxford: Blackwell, pp49–59.

Department for Children, Schools and Families (DCSF) (2003) *Every Child Matters (ECM)*, Command Paper presented to HM Government, September 2003, Cd 5680. London: HMSO. Available online at www.every childmatters.gov.uk.

Department of Health (DH) (1999) *Royal Commission on Long Term Care*. Cm 4192–1. London: HMSO.

Department of Health (DH) (2000) *The NHS Plan: A plan for investment, a plan for reform*. London: HMSO.

Department of Health (DH) (2001) *The Essence of Care: Patient-focused benchmarking for health care practitioners* (revised 2003). London: HMSO.

Department of Health (DH) (2002a) *Liberating the Talents: Helping primary care trusts and nurses to deliver the NHS plan*. London: HMSO.

Department of Health (DH) (2002b) *Guidance on the Single Assessment Process for Older People*. HSC 2002/001,LAC. London: HMSO.

Department of Health (DH) (2004a) *The Knowledge and Skills Framework*. London: HMSO.

Department of Health (DH) (2004b) *Agenda for Change*. London: HMSO.

Department of Health (DH) (2004c) *Code of Practice for the International Recruitment of Healthcare Professionals*. Available online at www.dh.gov.uk/prod_consum_dh/groups/dh_digitalassets/0dh/0en/documents/digitalasset/dh_4097734.pdf.

Department of Health (DH) (2004d) *National Service Framework for Children, Young People and Maternity Services.* London: The Stationery Office.

Department of Health (DH) (2006) *Modernising Nursing Careers: Setting the direction.* London: HMSO.

Department of Health (DH) (2007a) *About the Chief Nursing Officer.* Available online at www.dh.gov.uk/en/Aboutus/Chiefprofessionalofficers/Chiefnursingofficer/DH_4000299 (accessed 23 June 2009).

Department of Health (DH) (2007b) *Global Health Partnerships: The UK contribution to health in developing countries.* London: The Stationery Office.

Department of Health (DH) (2008a) *Health is Global: A UK Government strategy 2008–13.* London: HMSO.

Department of Health (DH) (2008b) *High Quality Care for All: NHS next stage review final report* (Chair Lord Darzi of Denham), CM 7432. London: The Stationery Office.

Department of Health (DH) (2009) *Valuing People Now: A new three-year strategy for people with learning disabilities.* London: HMSO.

Department of Health and Social Security (DHSS) (1980) *Inequalities in Health : Report of a research working group chaired by Sir Douglas Black (The Black Report).* London: HMSO.

DiCenso, A and Cullum, N (1998) Implementing evidence based nursing: some misconceptions. *Evidence Based Nursing,* 1: 38–9.

Dougherty, L and Lister, S (2007) *The Royal Marsden Hospital Manual of Clinical Nursing Procedures,* 7th edition. London: Wiley-Blackwell.

Duffy, M (2001) A critique of cultural education in nursing. *Journal of Advanced Nursing,* 36: 487–95.

Edmond, CB (2001) A new paradigm for practice education. *Nurse Education Today,* 21: 251–9.

Ellis, P (2010) *Evidence-based Practice in Nursing.* Exeter: Learning Matters.

Eraut, M (1994) *Developing Professional Knowledge and Competence.* London: Falmer Press.

Etzioni, A (1969) *The Semi-Professions and Their Organisation.* London: Collier-Macmillan.

European Commission (EC) (1999) *Bologna Declaration.* Available online at ec.europa.eu/education/policies/educ/bologna/bologna.pdf (accessed May 2011).

European Commission (EC) (2007) *The Erasmus Programme Celebrates its 20th Anniversary.* Available online at ec.europa.eu/education/news/erasmus20_en.html (accessed May 2011).

European Resuscitation Council (ERC) (2010) *Basic Life Support (BLS) Guidelines.* Available online at www.erc.edu/index.php/guidelines_download.

European Resuscitation Council (2010) *Guidelines.* Available to download from www.erc.edu (last accessed, May 2011).

European Union (EU) (1987) *1980–1989 The Changing Face of Europe.* Available online at europa.eu/abc/history/1980-1989/index_en.htm (accessed May 2011).

European Union (EU) (2005) Directive 2005/36/EC of the European Parliament and of the Council of 7 September 2005 on the Recognition of Professional Qualifications. *Official Journal of the European Union,* 30 September 2005, Brussels.

European Union (EU) (2009) *Panorama of the European Union.* Luxemborg: EU Publications Office.

Fletcher, K (2007) Image: changing how women nurses think about themselves. Literature review. *Journal of Advanced Nursing,* 58(3): 207–13.

Ford, P, McCormack, B, Wills, T, Dewing, J (2000) Defining the boundaries: Nursing and personal care. *Nursing Standard,* 15(3), October: 43–5.

Fradd, E (2010) Gradually graduating to graduateness: the impact of nursing becoming a graduate profession. Conference paper presented at the University of Nottingham, 20 July.

Gass, J, McKie, A, Smith, I, Brown, A and Addo, M (2007) An examination of the scope and purpose of education in mental health nursing. *Nurse Education Today*, 27: 588–96.

Gerrish, K (2000) Still fumbling along? A comparative study of the newly qualified nurse's perception of the transition from student to qualified nurse. *Journal of Advanced Nursing*, 32: 473–80.

Glendinning, C (2007) Improving equity and sustainability in UK funding for long term care: lessons from Germany. *Social Policy and Society*, 6 (3), July: 411–22.

Goodman, B and Clemow, R (2010) *Nursing and Collaborative Practice*, 2nd edition. Exeter: Learning Matters.

Gorton, V (2004) Individual student learning contracts can facilitate student overseas study opportunities, in Danaher, PA, Macpherson, C, Nouwens, F and Orr, D (eds) *Lifelong Learning: Whose responsibility and what is your contribution?: Proceedings of the 3rd International Lifelong Learning Conference*, Yeppoon, Queensland, Australia, 13–16 June 2004. Rockhampton: Central Queensland University Press, pp1–12.

Greenhalgh, C, Roberts, J and Hill, I (1994) *The Interface between Junior Doctors and Nurses: A research study for the Department of Health*. Macclesfield: Greenhalgh and Co.

Hallam, J (1998) From angels to handmaidens: changing constructions of nursing's public image in post war Britain. *Nursing Inquiry*, 5: 32–42.

Hallett, C (2007) Editorial: A 'gallop' through history: nursing in a social context. *Journal of Clinical Nursing*, 16(3): 429.

Hardyman, R and Hickey, G (2001) What do newly-qualified nurses expect from preceptorship? Exploring the perspective of the preceptee. *Nurse Education Today*, 21: 58–64.

Hartigan, I, Murphy, S, Flynn, AV and Walshe, N (2010) Acute nursing episodes which challenge graduates' competence: Perceptions of registered nurses. *Nurse Education in Practice*, 10(5): 291–7.

Health and Safety Executive (HSE) (1995) *Reporting of Injuries, Diseases and Dangerous Occurrences Regulations* (RIDDOR). London: HSE. Available online at www.hse.gov.uk/riddor/riddor.htm (accessed May 2011).

Henderson, V (1966) *The Nature of Nursing: A definition and its implications for practice and education*. New York: Macmillan.

HM Government (1946) *National Health Service Act*. London: HMSO.

HM Government (1968) *Medicines Act*. London: HMSO.

HM Government (1971) *Misuse of Drugs Act*. London: HMSO.

HM Government (1985) *Misuse of Drugs Regulations SI 1985/2066*. London: HMSO.

HM Government (1989) *The Children Act*. London: HMSO.

HM Government (1998) *The Data Protection Act*. London: HMSO.

HM Government (2002) *The Nursing and Midwifery Order 2001(SI 2002/253)*. London: HMSO.

HM Government (2004) *The Children Act*. London: The Stationery Office.

Hockenbury, M and Wilson, D (2007) *Wong's Nursing Care of Infants and Children*, 8th edition. New York: Mosby.

Hole, J (2005) *The Newly Qualified Nurse's Survival Guide*. Oxford: Radcliffe.

Howatson-Jones, L (2010) *Reflective Practice in Nursing*. Exeter: Learning Matters.

International Council of Nurses (ICN) (2010) Definition of Nursing. Geneva: ICN. Available online at www.icn.ch/about-icn/definition-of-nursing (accessed May 2011).

Jackson, C (2005) The experience of a good day: a phenomenological study to explain a good day as experienced by a newly qualified RN. *Accident and Emergency Nursing*, 13: 110–21.

James, H and Trauner, DA (1985) The Glasgow Coma Scale, in James, H, Annas, N and Perkins, R (eds) *Brain Insults in Infants and Children*. Orlando, FL: Grune and Stratton, pp179–82.

Jinks, AM and Bradley, E (2004) Angel, handmaiden, battleaxe or whore? A study which examines changes in newly recruited student nurses' attitudes to gender and nursing stereotypes. *Nurse Education Today*, 24(2): 121–7.

Kallisch, BJ and Kallisch, PA (1983) Improving the image of nursing. *American Journal of Nursing*, 83(1): 48–55.

Keenan, J (1999) A concept analysis of autonomy. *Journal of Advanced Nursing*, 29(3): 556–62.

Kelsey, J and McEwing, G (2008) *Clinical Skills in Child Health Practice*. Edinburgh: Churchill Livingstone.

Kennedy, I (2001) *Learning from Bristol: The report of the public inquiry into children's heart surgery at the Bristol Royal Infirmary 1984–1995*, CM 5207. London: HMSO.

Kenworthy, N, Snowley, G and Gilling, C (eds) (2002) *Common Foundation Studies in Nursing*. Edinburgh: Churchill Livingstone.

Kevern, J and Webb, C (2004) Mature women's experiences in pre-registration nurse education. *Journal of Advanced Nursing*, 45(3): 297–306.

Khomeiran, R, Yekta, ZP, Kiger, AM and Ahmadi, F (2006) Professional competence: factors described by nurses as influencing their development. *International Nursing Review*, 53: 66–72.

Kim, KH (2007) Clinical competence among senior nursing students after their preceptorship experiences. *Journal of Professional Nursing*, 23(6): 369–75.

Knowles, MS, Holton, EF and Swanson, RA (1998) *The Adult Learner*, 5th edition. Woburn, MA: Butterworth-Heinemann.

Kramer, M (1974) *Reality Shock: Why nurses leave nursing*. St Louis, MO: CV Mosby.

Laming, Lord (2009) *The Protection of Children In England: A progress report*. London: The Stationery Office.

Leach, MJ (2008) Planning: a necessary step in clinical care. *Journal of Clinical Nursing*, 17(13): 1728–34.

Liaschenko, J and Peter E (2004) Nursing ethics and conceptualisations of nursing: profession, practice and work. *Journal of Advanced Nursing*, 46(5): 488–95.

Lofmark, A, Smide, B and Wikblad, K (2006) Competence of newly-graduated nurses: a comparison of the perceptions of qualified nurses and students. *Journal of Advanced Nursing*, 53(6): 721–8.

Lowes, R, Peters, H and Turner, M (2004) *The International Student's Guide*. London: Sage.

Maben, J and Macleod Clark, J (1998) Project 2000 diplomates' perceptions of their experiences of transition from student to staff nurse. *Journal of Clinical Nursing*, 7: 145–53.

Maben, J, Latter, S and Macleod Clark, J (2006) The theory–practice gap: impact of professional–bureaucratic work conflict on newly-qualified nurses. *Journal of Advanced Nursing* 55(4): 465–77.

Maben, J, Latter, S and Macleod Clark, J (2007) The sustainability of ideals, values and the nursing mandate: evidence from a longitudinal qualitative study *Nursing Inquiry* 14(2): 99–113.

Macdonald, H (2007) Relational ethics and advocacy in nursing: literature review. *Journal of Advanced Nursing*, 57(2): 119–26.

McHale, J and Tingle, J (2007) *Law and Nursing*, 3rd edition. Philadelphia, PA: Butterworth-Heinemann-Elsevier.

Macintosh, C (1997) A historical study of men in nursing. *Journal of Advanced Nursing*, 26(2): 232–6.

McKenna, H (1997) *Nursing Theories and Models*. London: Routledge.

McKenna, H and Slevin, O (2008) *Vital Notes for Nurses: Nursing models, theories and practice*. Chichester: Blackwells.

Mallik, M, Hall, C and Howard, D (eds) (2009) *Nursing Knowledge and Practice: A decision making approach*, 3rd edition. Edinburgh: Elsevier.

Marriner-Tomey, A and Alligood, MR (eds) (2006) *Nursing Theorists and their Work*, 6th edition. St Louis, MO: Mosby.

MENCAP (2004) *Treat Me Right: Better healthcare for people with a learning disability*. London: MENCAP.

MENCAP (2008) *Death By Indifference: Following up on the* Treat Me Right *report*. London: MENCAP.

Mooney, M (2007) Facing registration: the expectations and the unexpected. *Nurse Education Today*, 27: 840–7.

Mosby (2009) *Mosby's Medical Dictionary*, 8th edition. London: Elsevier/Mosby.

National Health Service Institute for Innovation and Improvement (NHSIII) (2008) *The Productive Ward: Releasing time to care* (web-based package). Available online at www.institute.nhs.uk/quality_and_value/productivity_series/the_productive_series.htm.

National Health Service Litigation Authority (NHSLA) (2005) *Mental Health and Learning Disability Clinical Risk Management*. London: NHSLA.

National Health Service Modernisation Agency (2003) *New Ways of Working*. London: Department of Health.

National Institute for Health and Clinical Excellence/Royal College of Nursing (NICE/RCN) (2005) *Quick Reference Guide: The prevention and treatment of pressure ulcers*. Available online at www.nice.org.uk/nice media/pdf/CG029quickrefguide.pdf (accessed 28 June 2009).

Nightingale, F (1859) *Notes on Hospitals*. London: Longman.

Nightingale, F (1860) *Notes on Nursing: What it is and what it is not*. New York: Appleton.

Nolan, M and Caldock, K (1996) Assessment: identifying the barriers to good practices. *Health & Social Care in the Community*, 4(2): 77–85.

Nursing and Midwifery Council (NMC) (2002) *Records and Record Keeping*. London: NMC.

Nursing and Midwifery Council (NMC) (2004a) *Standards of Proficiency for Pre-registration Nursing Education*. London: NMC.

Nursing and Midwifery Council (NMC) (2004b) *Code of Professional Conduct: Standards of conduct, performance and ethics*. London: NMC.

Nursing and Midwifery Council (NMC) (2006) *Preceptorship Guidelines*, NMC circular 21/2006. London: NMC.

Nursing and Midwifery Council (NMC) (2008a) *Code of Professional Conduct: Standards of conduct, performance and ethics*, revised version. London: NMC.

Nursing and Midwifery Council (NMC) (2008b) *A Review of Pre-registration Nursing Education: Report of consultation findings for the Nursing and Midwifery Council*. London: NMC (prepared by Alpha Research).

Nursing and Midwifery Council (NMC) (2009a) *Guidance on Professional Conduct for Nursing and Midwifery Students.* London: NMC.

Nursing and Midwifery Council (NMC) (2009b) *NMC Review of Pre-registration Nursing Education*, Bulletin 1, February. Available online at www.nmc-uk.org.

Nursing and Midwifery Council (NMC) (2009c) *Record Keeping: Guidance for nurses and midwives.* London: NMC.

Nursing and Midwifery Council (NMC) (2010) *Standards of Competence for Pre-registration Nursing Education.* London: NMC.

O'Connor, SE, Pearce, J, Smith, RL, Voegeli, D and Walton, P (2001) An evaluation of the clinical performance of newly qualified nurses: a competency based assessment. *Nurse Education Today*, 21: 559–68.

Office for National Statistics (ONS) (2000) *The United Kingdom Standard Occupational Classification System.* London: HMSO.

Orem, DE (1985) *Nursing: Concepts of practice*, 2nd edition. New York: McGraw Hill.

Orem, DE (2001) *Nursing: Concepts of practice*, 6th edition. St Louis, MO: Mosby.

O'Shea, M and Kelly, B (2007) The lived experiences of newly qualified nurses on clinical placement during the first six months following registration in the Republic of Ireland. *Journal of Clinical Nursing*, 16: 1534–42.

Papadopoulos, I (ed.) (2006) *Transcultural Health and Social Care: Development of culturally competent practitioners.* Edinburgh: Elsevier/Churchill Livingstone.

Parsons, T (1951) *The Social System.* London: Routledge and Kegan Paul.

Payne, D (2000) New year, new image. *Nursing Times*, 96(1): 14–15.

Peplau, HE (1952) *Interpersonal Relations in Nursing.* New York: GP Putnam's Sons.

Pesut, B and Johnson, J (2008) Reinstating the 'Queen': understanding philosophical inquiry in nursing. *Journal of Advanced Nursing*, 61(1): 115–21.

Pratt, S (2001) Competent on qualifying? *Paediatric Nursing*, 13(9): 32–3.

Ramritu, P and Barnard A (2001) New nurse graduates' understanding of competence. *International Nursing Review*, 48: 47–57.

Red Spider Ltd (2004) The desired core values of nursing: analysis of the *Nursing Standard* workshop 1104. *Nursing Standard*, 19(30): 24.

Reed, S (2011) *Successful Professional Portfolios for Nursing Students.* Exeter: Learning Matters.

Riddick, E (2010) *Mental Health Nursing: Job description and activities.* Available online at ww2.prospects. ac.uk/p/types_of_job/mental_health_nurse_job_description.jsp (accessed May 2011).

Roper, N, Logan, WW and Tierney, AJ (1980) *The Elements of Nursing.* Edinburgh: Churchill Livingstone.

Roper, N, Logan, WW and Tierney, AJ (eds) (1983) *Using a Model for Nursing.* Edinburgh: Churchill Livingstone.

Roper, N, Logan, WW and Tierney, AJ (1990) *The Elements of Nursing*, 3rd edition. Edinburgh: Churchill Livingstone.

Roper, N, Logan, WW and Tierney, AJ (2000) *The Roper–Logan–Tierney Model of Nursing: Based on activities of living.* Edinburgh: Churchill Livingstone.

Ross, H and Clifford, K (2002) Research as a catalyst for change: the transition from student to Registered Nurse. *Journal of Clinical Nursing*, 11: 545–53.

Roy, C (1970) Adaptation: a conceptual framework for nursing. *Nursing Outlook*, 18(3): 42–5.

Roy, C (1976) *Introduction to Nursing: An adaptation model*. Englewood Cliffs, NJ: Prentice Hall.

Royal College of Nursing (RCN) (2003) *Defining Nursing*. London: RCN. Available online at www.rcn.org.uk/ (accessed May 2011).

Royal College of Nursing (2009) *Knowledge and Skills Framework and Appraisal Guidance for Members and Employers outside of the NHS*. London: RCN.

Rungapadiachy, DM; Madill, A and Gough, B (2006) How newly qualified mental health nurses perceive their role. *Journal of Psychiatric and Mental Health Nursing*, 13: 533–42.

Ryan, M and Twibell, RS (2002) Outcomes of a transcultural nursing immersion experience: confirmation of a dimensional matrix. *Journal of Transcultural Nursing*, 13(1): 30–9.

Scriven, A and Garman, S (2005) *Promoting Health Global Perspectives*. Basingstoke: Palgrave Macmillan.

Smith, F (1995) *Children's Nursing in Practice: The Nottingham model*. Oxford: Blackwell Science.

Spouse, J (2000) An impossible dream? Images of nursing held by pre-registration students and their effects on sustaining motivation to become nurses. *Journal of Advanced Nursing*, 32 (3): 730–9.

Standing, M (2011) *Clinical Judgement and Decision-making for Nursing Students*. Exeter: Learning Matters.

Sumner, WG (1906) What is critical thinking? Cited by The Critical Thinking Community. Available online at www.criticalthinking.org/aboutCT/sumnersDefinitionCT.cfm (accessed 23 June 2009).

Takase, M, Kershaw, E and Burt, L (2002) Does public image of nursing matter? *Journal of Professional Nursing*, 18(4): 196–205.

Thompson, L and Hall, C (2007) Exploring student nurses' educational needs in relation to end-of-life care in children. *Journal of Children's and Young People's Nursing*, 1(6): 281–6.

Timmins, F and Horan, P (2007) A critical analysis of the potential contribution of Orem's (2001) self-care deficit nursing theory to contemporary coronary care nursing practice. *European Journal of Cardiovascular Nursing* 6(1): 32–9.

Tones, K and Green, J (2004) *Health Promotion: Planning and strategies*. London: Sage.

Tones, K and Tilford, S (2001) *Health Promotion: Effectiveness, efficiency, and equity*, 3rd edition. Cheltenham: Nelson Thornes.

Turner, M and Thomas, B (2006) *Talking with Children and Young People about Death and Dying*. London: Jessica Kingsley.

Wanless, D (2002) *Securing our Future Health: Taking a long-term view*. London: The Stationery Office.

Williamson, GR, Jenkinson, T and Proctor-Childs. T (2010) *Contexts of Contemporary Nursing*, 2nd edition. Exeter: Learning Matters.

World Health Organization (WHO) (1946) *Preamble to the Constitution of the World Health Organization as adopted by the International Health Conference*, New York, 19 June–22 July 1946; signed on 22 July 1946 by the representatives of 61 States (Official Records of the World Health Organization, no. 2, p. 100) and entered into force on 7 April 1948. Geneva: WHO. Available online at www.who.int/suggestions/faq/en/ (accessed 23 June 2009).

World Health Organization (WHO) (1948) *Official Records of the World Health Organization*, no. 2. Geneva: WHO.

World Health Organization (WHO) (2007) *Annual Report: A Safer Future: Global public health security in the 21st century.* Geneva: WHO.

World Health Organization (WHO) (2008) *Annual Report: Primary Health Care: 'Now more than ever'.* Geneva: WHO.

World Health Organization (WHO) (2011) *About WHO.* Available online at www.who.int/about/en (accessed April 2011).

Wright, K (2005) Care planning: an easy guide for nurses. *Nursing & Residential Care*, 7: 71–3.

Index

A

absence, sickness 47–8
access
  to health records 79
  to healthcare 67
accountability 12, 32–3, 41, 78–9, 91–2, 126
Activities of Living Model 59–60, 64, 81–2, 84
Adaptation Model 58
adult nursing 171–9, 181
advocacy 20–1, 62–3, 150–1, 180
AEIs *see* approved education institutes
Agenda for Change 18–19, 29, 137
AGREE Collaboration 90
Andrews, Margaret 104
'angel' nursing stereotype 37
antibiotics, resistance to 20–1, 68
Anxiety and Depression Scale 83–4
appearance 42–3
applications, employment 133–4
  interviews 134–5
  post-interview 136
approved education institutes (AEIs) 99, 107, 108,
    113, 115
assessment, elective experiences 115
assessment of patients 75, 76–8, 125
  consent/confidentiality 78–9, 80–1, 95–6, 158
  measurement tools 82–4
  observation 79–82
  SOAPIER tool 75–6
autonomy 15–17, 28, 33

B

'battle-axe' stereotype 38
Beasley, Christine 7
Beauchamp, Tom 33
Becker's Health Belief Model 58, 65, 67
beliefs about nursing 53–4, 69–70
beneficence 33
BILD *see* British Institute of Learning Disabilities
Black, Beth Perry 56
Black Report 106
Bolam Test 91–2
Bologna Process 109
Boyle, Joyceen 104
Bradley, Eleanor 39
Bridges, Jacqueline 36–7
Bristol Royal Infirmary Inquiry 43

British Institute of Learning Disabilities (BILD)
  152
Brookfield, Stephen 22
BUNAC 114
Burton, William 117

C

C. diff. 20, 68
Caldock, Kerry 81
care delivery 90–2
  quality of 32–3, 127–9
  see also 'nursing process'
care environment 20–1, 67–9
career opportunities
  adult nursing 176–7
  children's nursing 160
  learning disability (LD) nursing 151–2
  mental health nursing 168–9
Centre for Evidence Based Medicine (CEBM) 90
character *see* conduct, professional
Chief Nursing Officer (CNO) 7
Children Act (1989) 81
children's nursing 153–61, 180–1
  parental responsibility 81
Childress, James 33
Chitty, Kay Kittrell 56
Citizens Advice Bureau, *Advice Guide* 71
civil law 11, 13
clinical skills 125–6
Clostridium difficile (C. diff.) 20, 68
CNO *see* Chief Nursing Officer
Cochrane Collaboration 90
Code of Practice for the International Recruitment of
    Healthcare Professionals 101
Code of Professional Conduct (NMC) 32, 41–2
collaboration 17–20
communication 42–3, 94
  children's nursing 155–7
compassion 31
competence 10–11, 91–2
  scope and quality 32
  see also professionalism; skills
conduct, professional 33–5, 47–8, 91–2
  Code of Professional Conduct (NMC) 32, 41–2
  see also images of nurses/nursing
confidentiality/consent 78–9, 95–6
  children's nursing 80–1, 158

consciousness, Glasgow Coma Scale 83
consent *see* confidentiality/consent
continuing professional development *see* lifelong
    learning
contracts of employment 136
cover letters, employment 133
Cox, Chris 12
Crawford, Doreen 159
criminal law 12, 13
criminal offences 48
Critical Appraisal Skills Programme 90
critical thinking 21–3
Crombie, Iain 90
Cullum, Nicky 89
cultural awareness 105, 110
culture 102–3
    transcultural nursing 94–8
culture shock, elective experiences 113–14
curricula, internationalising 108
CVs 133–4

D
Darzi Inquiry 63
data, objective/subjective 76, 80
Data Protection Act (2000) 79, 96
death and dying 64, 125–6, 159
deductive thinking 56. 70
Defining Nursing (RCN) 8–9, 71
degree-level education 43–6
delegation 91, 127, 140
Department of Health (DH) 7
    and global health 100, 101, 106
depression, Hospital Anxiety and Depression
    Scale 83–4
DiCenso, Alba 89
disabilities
    learning disability (LD) nursing 145–53,
      180
    mental health nursing 13, 59, 62, 161–71
    reasonable adjustments 34
disclosure *see* confidentiality/consent
'doctor's handmaiden' stereotype 38–9
documentation *see* record keeping
'doers', nurses as 44, 60–2, 69
domains of practice 30
dress, job interviews 135

E
elderly care
    debates on funding 19
    see also adult nursing

elective experiences 105, 107–8, 108–9,
    117–18
    assessment of 115, 116
    benefits 110–11
    challenges/concerns 112–13
    and culture 110, 113–15
    portfolio development 110–11, 115–16
emergency situations 68, 121–2, 126
employment 130–1, 136–7
    applications 133–6, 141
    financial matters 137–9
    job descriptions 132–3, 136
    see also career opportunities
empowerment *see* patient empowerment
environment for care 20–1, 67–9
equal opportunities, employment 135
Equality and Human Rights Commission 34
ERASMUS Scheme 108, 112
Eraut, Michael 32
Essence of Care benchmarks 68
Essential Skills Clusters (ESCs) 3, 11
ethical principles 33
European Resuscitation Council (ERC) 58,
    68–9
European Union (EU) 101
    legal requirements 14
    student exchanges 108–9
European Working Time Directive 15
evaluation, 'nursing process' 75, 92–3, 95
Every Child Matters 161
evidence-based practice 88–90
    critical thinking 21–3
exchange programmes *see* elective experiences

F
facilitators, nurses as 61, 66–7
feminism 38
finance
    employment 137–9
    see also funding
First World War 16
fitness to practise 30, 34, 47–8
Fradd, Dame Elizabeth 45
funding
    elective experiences 112
    healthcare 17–18, 19, 57

G
gender
    male nursing students 40
    stereotypes of nurses/nursing 36–41

Glasgow Coma Scale (GCS) 83
'global health' concept 99–102
    and nurse education 1–2
    see also transcultural nursing
Global Health Partnerships 101, 106
globalisation 100
graduate education 43–6

H
HAIs *see* hospital-acquired infections
Hall, Carol 159
HCSWs *see* healthcare support workers
'health' concept 54, 57–60, 63–4
    and the care environment 20–1, 67–9
    definitions 64, 105
    and patient empowerment 62, 62–3, 65–7
Health and Safety Executive (HSE) 13
Health Belief Model 58, 65, 67
Health is Global strategy 100–1
Health Rights Information Scotland (HRIS) 71
healthcare support workers (HCSWs) 127
Henderson, Virginia 60, 64
holidays *see* travel
homeostatic balance 69
Horan, Paul 70–1
hospital-acquired infections (HAIs) 20–1, 68
Hospital Anxiety and Depression Scale 83–4
HRIS *see* Health Rights Information Scotland
HSE *see* Health and Safety Executive
'hygiene' concept 67–8

I
ICN *see* International Council of Nurses
identification of nurses 43
images of nurses/nursing 35–6
    and degree-level education 43–6
    importance of 41–3
    specific stereotypes 36–41
    see also conduct, professional
implementation, 'nursing process' 75, 87–8, 92
incidents, reporting 13, 24
induction programmes 125, 130
inductive thinking 56, 70
inequalities, global healthcare 105–6
information
    analysis 84
    sharing 94
    see also assessment of patients;
        confidentiality/consent; record keeping
*Integrated Multi-agency Care Pathways for Children with
    Life-threatening and Life-limiting Conditions* 64

integrity 31, 33
    see also conduct, professional
International Council of Nurses (ICN) 9–10
interviews
    employment 134–5
    patients 80–2

J
Jinks, Annette 39
job seeking *see* employment
justice 33

K
Kennedy Report 43
Kenworthy, Neil 103, 104
Knowledge and Skills Framework (KSF) 19, 29,
    137

L
language acquisition 112
law *see* legal requirements
Leach, Matthew 85, 86
leadership skills 126–7
learning disability (LD) nursing 145–53, 180
    see also mental health nursing
legal requirements 11–13, 32–3
    Bolam Test 91–2
    European 14
Liaschenko, Joan 28
lifelong learning 110–11, 129
    Knowledge and Skills Framework 19, 29, 137
Logan, Winifred, Activities of Living Model
    59–60, 64, 81–2, 84
Lowes, Ricky 113
Lucy, Gary 66

M
MacDonald, Hannah 151
male nursing students 40
'man' concept 54, 57–8
management skills 126–7
matrons, stereotypes of 38
mature students 40, 46, 112
McHale, Jean 12
McKenna, Hugh 56
media
    access to 67
    images of nurses 35, 37, 38, 39
medicines administration 125
men in nursing 40
MENCAP 150–1

Mental Health Alliance 170
mental health nursing 13, 59, 62, 161–71
    see also learning disability (LD) nursing
mentoring/mentors 12, 32, 40, 121–2, 127, 134
    preceptorship 129–30, 141
'ministering angel' stereotype 37
mobility/movement, health workers 100, 101, 109
    see also elective experiences
motivation, elective experiences 110
MRSA 20, 68
multiculturalism 110, 115
    see also transcultural nursing

N
name badges 43
National Health Service *see* NHS
National Institute for Health and Clinical
    Excellence (NICE) 90
National Insurance 139
National Occupational Standards (NOS) 18
'naughty nurse' stereotype 38
negligence 12
    Bolam test 91–2
next of kin 80–1
NHS (National Health Service) 15, 35, 45, 175
    Agenda for Change 18–19, 29, 137
    wages and pay 137–8
NHS and You, The 71
NHS Institute for Innovation and Improvement
    (NHSIII) 175–6
NICE 90
Nightingale, Florence 20, 37, 67–8, 70
NMC *see* Nursing and Midwifery Council
Nolan, Mike 81
non-maleficence 33
non-medical prescribing 18
Northern Ireland 34
NOS *see* National Occupational Standards
Nottingham Model 70
nurse education
    degree-level 43–6
    and 'global health' 102
    see also elective experiences
'nursing' concept 54–5, 57–60
    core values 31–2
    definitions 7–13
    history 14–21, 37
    philosophy 55–7
    theories 54–7, 69–70, 70–1
    see also images of nurses/nursing; Nightingale,
        Florence; 'nursing process'

Nursing and Midwifery Council (NMC) 10–11,
    14, 29–30, 33–4, 47
    the *Code* 32, 41–2
    registration 136
    standards and ESCs 3, 11, 30, 99
nursing process 74–5
    care delivery 90–2
    confidentiality/consent 78–9, 80–1, 95–6, 158
    evaluation 75, 92–3, 95
    implementation 75, 87–8, 92
    planning/goals 75, 85–7
    see also assessment of patients; roles and
        responsibilities
Nursing Standard, Nursing the Future campaign 31

O
objective data 76, 80
observation, patients 79–82
ontology 55–6
Orem, Dorothea, Self-care Deficit Theory 58–9,
    61–2, 66, 70–1
organisational policy 127–9

P
pain, indicators of 84
palliative care 64
    see also death and dying
Papadopoulos, Irena 104
parents, children's nursing 81, 156–7
parliamentary debates, elderly care 19
Parsons, Talcott 65
patient-centred care 75–6
patient dependency 126
patient empowerment 62, 62–3, 65–7
patients' rights 33, 67
pay structures *see* Agenda for Change
pensions 139
Peplau, Hildegard 59, 62, 63
Perceptions Forum 170
Peter, Elizabeth 28
philosophy of nursing 55–7
planning/goals, 'nursing process' 75, 85–7
policy, organisational 127–9
political contexts 16–17
portfolio development 110–11, 115–16
power relations, nurses/doctors 38–9
Prague Declaration 109
preceptorship 129–30
prescribing, non-medical 18
presentations, employment 135
pressure sores, Waterlow Score 83

Primary Health Care (WHO) 68
private sector pay 138
'problem', use of term 84
professionalism 29–32
   and the student nurse 32–5
   see also conduct, professional; image of
      nurses/nursing
professionals, nurses as 27–9
   degree-level education 43–6

Q
qualification(s) 43–6
   concerns/problems 121–4, 140
   registration 136
   required hours 14
   see also employment; roles and responsibilities;
      support mechanisms
quality of care 32–3, 127–9

R
RCN *see* Royal College of Nursing
Real Gap 114
reasonable adjustments, disabled students 34
record keeping 94–5, 96
   see also assessment of patients
references, employment 134
registration, NMC 136
regulators of nursing 10–11
research, newly qualified nurses 123–4
responsibility *see* accountability; roles and
    responsibilities
resuscitation 58, 68–9
RIDDOR (Reporting of Injuries, Diseases and
    Dangerous Occurrence Regulations) 13
rights of patients 33, 67
roles and responsibilities 60
   newly qualified nurses 124–9
   nurse as advocate 20–1, 62–3, 150–1, 180
   nurse as 'doer/intervener' 44, 60–2, 69
   see also 'nursing process'
Roper, Nancy, Activities of Living Model 59–60,
    64, 81–2, 84
rotational posts 130
Roy, Callista, Adaptation Model 58, 69
Royal College of Nursing (RCN) 8–9, 71

S
Safer Future, A (WHO) 100
safety of environment 20–1
scope, competence 32
Self-care Deficit Theory 58–9, 61–2, 66, 70–1

sexual stereotypes, nurses 38, 40
'sick' role 65–6
sickness absences 47–8
Single Assessment Process (SAP) for Older
    People 77
skills
   adult nursing 171–4
   children's nursing 154–8
   clinical 125–6
   leadership/management 126–7
   learning disability nursing 146–9
   mental health nursing 162–5
skills initiatives
   Essential Skills Clusters 3, 11
   Knowledge and Skills Framework 19, 29,
    137
   Skills for Health 18
Slevin, Oliver 56
SMART concept 85
SOAPIER assessment tool 75–6
social contexts 16–17
'society' concept 54, 57–60
specialist units 125
Spouse, Jenny 39
standards, NMC 3, 30, 99
stereotypes *see* images of nurses/nursing
student exchanges *see* elective experiences
subjective data 76, 80
suffragette movement 16
Sumner, William Graham 21–2
supernumerary status 91
support mechanisms 129–30, 141
   mentoring/mentors 12, 32, 40, 121–2,
    127, 134
   supervision 32, 40, 77, 90–2, 126–7, 130,
    137

T
tax 139
teamwork 31, 126–7
terminal illness *see* death and dying
theories of nursing 54–7, 69–70, 70–1
Thomas, Bob 159
Thompson, Lucy 159
Tierney, Alison, Activities of Living Model 59–60,
    64, 81–2, 84
Timmins, Fiona 70–1
Tingle, John 12
tools for nursing 74–6
   see also 'nursing process'
trade unions 9, 139

transcultural nursing 103–7
   see also elective experiences; 'global health' concept
travel 110, 114
   see also elective experiences
Turner, Mary 159

V
values, nursing 53–7, 104
Valuing People Now 153
versatility 31
Victorian nursing students 37

W
Wanless Report 29
Waterlow Score 83
Way, Colin 159
WHO *see* World Health Organization
women *see* images of nurses/nursing
work experience, global *see* elective
   experiences
World Health Organization (WHO) 9, 68,
   100, 106
   definition of 'health' 64, 105